ABOUT THE AUTHOR
Kurt W. Donsbach, D.C., N.D., Ph.D.

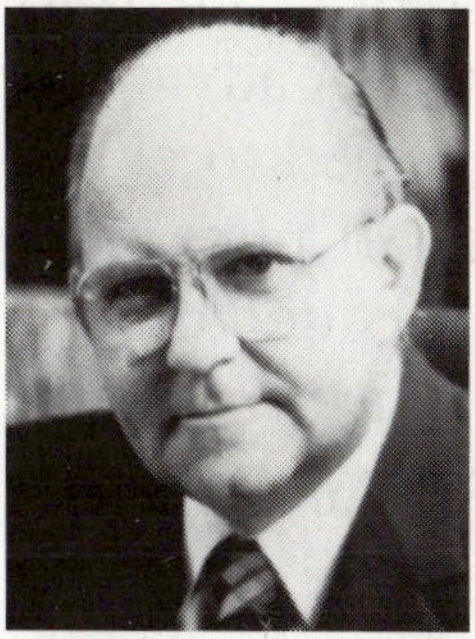

"Health is a frame of mind, a matter of attitude, of eating, and proper nutritional supplements," says one of America's foremost nutritionists and health care educators. "This nation is preoccupied with disease," he continues, "and not with health factors that bring about a complete and perfect function of all organs."

Coming from a rural background, Dr. Donsbach began his career in the healing arts as a chiropractic physician specializing in the treatment of arthritic and rheumatoid disorders. Later on he accepted a position with the famous Dr. Royal Lee, of the Lee Foundation for Nutritional Research, where he helped develop the foundation's theories on preventive organic medicine. He conceived one of the first Wholistic treatments of arthritis, treatment without pain killers.

Dr. Donsbach founded Donsbach University, School of Nutrition with overseas campuses in Israel, South Africa, Italy, Canada and Japan. He served as Chairman of the Board of Governors of the National Health Federation for 15 years and is director of Hospital Santa Monica and Institut Santa Monica, the two largest wholistic hospitals in the world. He is also a director of Agua Caliente, a health resort specializing in cell therapy, facial rejuvenation, weight reduction and detoxification. He has appeared on numerous radio and TV shows and had his own syndicated radio talk show airing daily for four years.

In addition to his bestselling book ***Embracing Wholistic Health***, Dr. Donsbach has authored over 40 publications on the subject of nutrition. His "Dr. *Donsbach Tells You What You Always Wanted To Know About...*" series has sold over 14 million copies.

Doctor, Educator, Scientist, Author, Lecturer, Consultant. With his entertaining sense of humor and his boundless energy, Dr. Donsbach sets forth to offer the key to healthier living to a nation that is thirsting for nutritional knowledge. With the help of Dr. H. Rudolph Alsleben, Dr. Donsbach has just opened ***The University of the Healing Arts,*** a Department of Education authorized home study program for those who truly wish to learn about the triune factors in healing – the body mind and spirit.

FOREWORD

This booklet is designed to inform those interested in avoiding the main cause of death as to what they can do before they suffer from advanced cardiovascular disease. It is not designed to either diagnose or treat this killer disease. It may offer the reader some real options to consider before partaking of the treatment of heart disease at the hands of the medical profession who, by their own admission, have failed miserably to halt the onslaught of cardiovascular disease.

The authors feel it is high time for the public to take matters into their own hands and do something positive to prevent diseases which all of us fear but which we seemingly cannot avoid.

Probably the most difficult of all the information presented in this booklet will be that which seems to indicate that there has been an unforgivable apathy on the part of organized medicine to recognize they may have made a mistake with their cholesterol mania and promoted not only the very disease they were trying to prevent (cardiovascular disease) but also increased the incidence of cancer by promoting the ingestion of highly unsaturated oils.

The authors only request that you read these documented facts and consider your own course.

KWD & WM

HEART DISEASE and STROKE

Heart disease and stroke are only a part of the condition known as cardiovascular disease. But they are the part of that complex disease which is an all too frequent cause of disability and/or death. The other signs of cardiovascular disease such as cold hands and cold feet, poor healing, cramping in the legs and toes, loss of memory, loss of energy, etc., are uncomfortable and limiting but do not directly cause death.

Prior to 1926, there was not one doctor in a thousand who had the faintest concept as to what myocardial infarction (heart attack) consisted of. After 1928 most doctors had heard of the disease, which they called coronary thrombosis, because they recognized the involvement of the coronary arteries. even though this was an unnamed disease before 1926, examination of the medical records indicated that the doctors were recording the symptoms of heart attack in their records, even in the late 1800's.

Drs. Finlayson (a pathologist) and Mackinnon (general practitioner) undertook a study to determine the actual incidence of cardiovascular disease over the years. Beginning in 1855, they reviewed physicians' records of patients. Knowing that myocardial infarction is now the cause of about 500,000 deaths every year, they were trying to find out if this disease was just misdiagnosed, or overlooked or whether it is, in fact, a disease peculiar to the mid 1900's.

The Mackinnon study took place in Yorkshire, England, a rural community with a very constant population of 22,000. His findings were as follows:

1855 - 1900 1 death per year per 22,000 pop.
1900 - 1925 5 deaths per year per 22,000 pop.
1925 - 1985 35 deaths per year per 22,000 pop.

Dr. Finlayson undertook his study in London reviewing hospital records and adjusting his numbers to reflect the amount of deaths per 22,000 population. An amazing correlation occurred: his statistics using urban residents as compared to a rural population in Yorkshire were identical! The death rates for the time periods outlined by Mackinnon were within less than a percentile the same as those found by Finlayson.

Here are some significant occurrences which may have been a factor in these statistics:

- 1910 - Machine-made cigarettes were marketed. 80 percent of the male population smoked.

- 1910 - White flour replaced whole wheat flour and everyone who had the money to purchase it used white rather than whole wheat flour.

We could legitimately theorize that these two changes in life style may have accounted for the increase of from 1 to 5 deaths per 22,000 population.

But the greatest jump in the death rate took place after 1925 and up to the present. There is one major change in lifestyle that could be relevant:

- In the late 1930's oils began to be used with increasing frequency by the homemakers of America. As a nation, we were a bit slow in taking up with margarine but rapid advances in technology made it a more acceptable, less expensive substitute for butter. Oils were rapidly replacing lard in the kitchen.

- In the 1950's cholesterol mania was born and everyone switched to highly refined, unsaturated oils, margarine and hydrogenated oil shortening.

Let us examine the significance of these happenings. In the late 1800's and early 1900's when the death rate from heart attack was practically zero (1 per year per 22,000 pop.), there was no margarine and no liquid polyunsaturated fats on the market. There was a little olive oil but its consumption was small and limited mostly to Italian families. People lived on a diet high in butter, cheese, eggs, meat and lard which today are touted as the cause of cardiovascular disease.

Today with a 35 time increase in deaths registered, we are told to use only unsaturated oils, margarine and shortening. Without question, evidence indicates that as hydrogenated margarine and shortening and liquid oils, such a corn oil, have replaced butter and lard in our diet, deaths from myocardial infarction have increased by 3500%! In Norway, during the German occupation, the Germans made off with half the margarine. During the war years, deaths in Norway from myocardial infarction decreased by one third. In the ten year postwar period, margarine consumption tripled. Is it a coincidence that deaths from myocardial infarction doubled in that 10 year period?

In the year 1949, no one in medicine was giving any thought to cholesterol and saturated fats as having anything to do with death from myocardial infarction. By the year 1957, cholesterol and saturated fats had **everything** to do with death from myocardial infarction according to popular opinion. The Prudent Diet was born and butter, cheese and lard were four letter words that became the convenient cause of the new epidemic - cardiovascular disease.

IRISH-BOSTON BROTHER STUDY

Two studies were designed to prove that butter and lard were bad and margarine and oils were good. Irish brothers, one of whom had immigrated to America, were used in this study. When this study was organized it was thought that the brothers in Ireland who did not have the benefit of the "good" margarines and oils, would be found to have far more deaths from myocardial infarction.

Surprise! What was found was that the deaths from myocardial infarction were significantly more frequent in the brothers living in Boston compared to their counterparts living in Ireland where butter and lard were the order of the day.

THE MALHOTRA STUDY

This study took place in India. A group of native Indians living near the city of Madras lived on a diet which was startlingly similar to the much touted Prudent Diet. They were vegetarians with very low levels of serum cholesterol, living mostly on rice. Their source of fats in the diet was peanut oil and a type of margarine made from this oil.

Dr. Malhotra was the physician for the Indian National Railway System. In studying these natives, he noted that there was a very high death rate from myocardial infarction. He compared their rate with a group of Indians living in the northern part of India near the city of Udaipur. These north Indians were perhaps the biggest butter eaters in the world. They ate butter as ghee, a semi-fluid butterfat from buffalo milk. Their serum cholesterols were considered to be high **but their southern vegetarian countrymen had 15 times as many deaths from myocardial infarction!**

One factor was noted about the butter eating Indians, they consumed a very large quantity of onions and garlic. The oil of onion and garlic contains methylallyl-trisulfide, a potent inhibitor of platelet aggregation. It prevents the formation of blood clots that so often are the cause of death in myocardial infarction. What did orthodox cardiologists have to say about the Irish Brothers and the Malhotra studies? Mainly they didn't say anything - they ignored them. This attitude could be summed up by: "Don't bother us with the facts at a time when we already have our minds made up."

There have been two possible explanations given as to how the vast increase in margarine and poly-unsaturated oil consumption has so greatly increased the death rate from heart attacks.

HYDROGENATION

When unsaturated oils are hydrogenated, which involves a process of forcing hydrogen gas into the oils, new and very unnatural substances are formed called "cis" and "trans" fatty acids. Because they have no useful purpose, these cis and trans fatty acids are real "clinkers" in our metabolism. But even worse, they act to inhibit other very necessary enzymes which help the body to form substances which reduces the "stickiness" of blood platelets. When blood platelets are sticky they tend to clump together, forming clots which easily plug up an artery already narrowed by plaque accumulation. In 1900 when death from heart attack was literally unknown, these unnatural fatty acids had not yet been introduced to our diet.

ANTIOXIDANT REMOVAL

When oils are processed from their source, another substance associated with all oils is separated out. This substance is the tocopherol family - we call it vitamin E. This vitamin is known for its anti-oxidant properties, which literally translated means that it prevents the changes associated with rancidity. Corn oil, from which the tocopherols have been removed, has been shown to be toxic to the hearts of animals. This corn oil-type damage is manifest by what are known as small areas of foci of degeneration in the heart muscle. Terence Anderson of the University of British Columbia teaches that these small degenerated areas in the heart muscle set off the arrhythmias (erratic heart beat) that are the final step to death from myocardial infarction.

An arrhythmic heart beats very weakly and rapidly which does not allow adequate blood to circulate to sustain life. In a great many cases of death from heart attack, initially there is a major blood clot in a coronary artery. This shuts off blood to a segment of the heart muscle which results in the actual death of many of these muscle cells. This is the "infarction" part of the condition. Lack of functional muscle cells creates the arrhythmia. Anderson holds that the muscle cell can be injured enough to cause arrhythmias without a blood clot closing off the coronary artery just by the damage done by vitamin E deficient corn oil ingestion.

In this modern day and age, we literally have a pandemic of myocardial infarction - and we have doctors telling patients that the eating of margarine and poly-unsaturated oils will prevent and cure myocardial infarction when there is an abundance of evidence that these cis and trans fatty acid substances are probably **the** major cause of death from myocardial infarction.

HOMOGENIZATION OF MILK

There was another environmental change that occurred in 1936 that may have had a great adverse effect on the death rate from myocardial infarction - the homogenization of milk. When a cow produces milk, a constituent called xanthine oxidase is found. Xanthine oxidase is an oxidizing enzyme and physically is a rather large particle. This large size prevents it from being absorbed through the tiny intestinal villi which pass substances from the gut into the blood stream. But after homogenization, these particles of xanthine oxidase can pass with ease because the process has changed them into tiny particles. This is true whether the milk is homogenized whole milk, skimmed or low fat.

The significance of this factor can be summed up by the work of Stephen Seely of the University of Manchester in England who did a world-wide study to find a single food associated with death from myocardial infarction. He found that there is a world-wide correlation between the drinking of liquid milk and heart disease but not with cheese consumption. The only difference between the two is that the milk used for drinking is homogenized and milk used for cheese is not.

Dr. Kurt Oster has done considerable research on xanthine oxidase and concludes that it is capable of causing significant harm to the wall of blood vessels and may even initiate the formation of plaque. This is quite believable because it is a substance that is totally unnatural to the internal environment of the body since its natural form could never enter into the blood stream.

WHITE OR WHEAT?

When everyone changed to white flour in the early 1900's, two factors which have a considerable impact on myocardial infarction were altered. One is that whole wheat bread is a reasonably good source of the tocopherols or vitamin E. The second is that whole wheat bread also contains considerable magnesium. We have discussed some of the anti-oxidant properties of vitamin E and their effect on preventing the rancidity changes in oils. It is interesting to note that the oil merchants remove the vitamin E and then sell it to vitamin manufacturers so that you can pay extra for something that was naturally present.

Before discussing the significance of magnesium on heart attacks, it should be pointed out that the Italian government banned the milling of white flour until after 1945 and their death rate from myocardial infarction did not catch up with that in the USA and England until 1947.

Terence Anderson, who did the study on corn oil, also noted that the Irish had a diet high in oatmeal which contains the necessary tocopherols and is rich in magnesium. You will remember the Irish Brothers study which indicated that a high consumption of butter and lard was not associated with a high rate of myocardial infarction.

MAGNESIUM

Finland is a small country world famous for its sturdy people. It is also infamous, called by some the "country of young widows" because of the premature deaths of its young men. Finland has the highest cardiovascular death rate in Europe. How so?

In 1957, a credible researcher, J. Kobayashi, first noted that the nature of drinking water might influence the death rates from heart disease. Finland is a soft water-drinking country. Later, investigations established that deaths in the United States from heart attacks in men 45 to 64 years old were significantly higher in states with soft water

Deaths from cerebrovascular accidents (strokes) followed a similar pattern. A study of three cities was undertaken which had different degrees of hardness in their water:

Lincoln, Nebraska	Hard Water
Washington, D.C.	Average Water
Savannah, Georgia	Soft Water

Death rates from heart attacks were compared:

Lincoln, Nebraska	300/1,000,000
Washington, D.C.	600/1,000,000
Savannah, Georgia	820/1,000,000

Although at one time it was considered that calcium was the protective factor in hard water, it is now known that magnesium is the protector. When you "soften" your water, you are taking out of your diet one of the most protective nutrients needed by man. In the early 1900's man had two fairly rich sources of this essential nutrient - whole grains and hard water. It is estimated that the average adult needs 6mg/kg of body weight of magnesium. This translates to about 500mg for a 185 pound person, but the national average consumption is less than one-half that amount.

A very important function of magnesium is that of maintaining normal heart rhythm even in the presence of low oxygen supply. Remember that arrhythmia is often the cause of death in myocardial infarction.

We really should bring in the aspirin studies at this time. All of us have been exposed to the great media event in 1989 which heralded aspirin as the shining new weapon against heart attack. If you know the true facts of this research, your thinking may be a little different. In the 1970's two studies were done in England and one in the USA which indicated that aspirin was worthless in preventing heart attacks. In 1989 another test was reported from England and one from the USA.

In the test in England, the doctors participating took aspirin and nothing else and there was no benefit note. In the USA the doctors took Bufferin, which contains aspirin and magnesium carbonate and magnesium oxide. There was a notable reduction in first-time heart attacks in the American study, but interestingly, no reduction in total death rate.

James A. Landauer of the Electrolyte Laboratories of Denver commented on these two tests. Landauer cited the many benefits of magnesium as the active factor:

a. Reduces platelet adhesion
b. Acts as an anticoagulant
c. Prolongs clotting time
d. Stimulates fibrinolytic activity
e. Is a powerful vasodilator
f. Facilitates release of prostacyclin

It thus becomes increasingly apparent that magnesium is a nutrient that everyone who is interested in their good health must be very aware of.

SUMMARY TO THIS POINT

1. Don't smoke
2. Use whole grains rather than refined
3. Don't ever use margarine
4. Don't ever use polyunsaturated oils
5. Stay away from homogenized milk
6. Do use butter
7. Do use garlic and onions
8. Use supplemental magnesium

CHELATION

What if someone told you that your case of severe hardening of the arteries need not lead to coronary bypass surgery or heart attack?

What if someone told you a safe, effective, tested, legal, non-surgical treatment exists which seems to be able to remove agents blocking blood flow in your arteries without side-effects?

And what if someone told you your heart specialist may not have even heard of the treatment and would be reluctant to prescribe it even if he had?

You would be amazed and perplexed, right? Well, if you plan to read further, you might want to sit down.

More than one million people die annually in this country from heart attacks. Fifty-five percent of all Americans who die of disease each year have an underlying case of atherosclerosis or hardening of the arteries.

A major remedy for arterial blockage is to transplant a vein or artery from the leg to bypass clogged portions of arteries in the heart. The operation, known as coronary bypass surgery, has a one to four percent mortality rate within two years. It costs a minimum of $50,000 and the costs may go well over $100,000 if everything doesn't go smoothly.

Life Style as a Factor

Due mainly to stress, diet and habits like smoking, drinking and taking in too many of society's pollutants, many modern Americans develop blockage of their arteries constricting blood flow and leading to poor circulation, senility, stroke, and ultimately heart attack and death. The material which blocks blood vessels builds up over 40 or 50 years and is comprised of fats, collagen, cholesterol and muscle tissue all bonded together by calcium. This blockage is known as **plaque.**

There are now two processes which can reverse or reduce atherosclerosis. These processes are called chelation therapy - oral and intravenous. Miraculous? Read on.

Heart Disease

Heart disease and stroke cause more deaths each year than all other causes of death combined, including cancer, accidents, pneumonia and influenza, diabetes and all other causes.

Heart Disease	1,000,000 plus deaths
Cancer	400,000 plus deaths
Accidents	100,000 plus deaths
Pneumonia & Flu	60,000 deaths
Diabetes	30,000 plus deaths
All others	300,000 plus deaths

The Number One Killer strikes nearly half its victims in the prime time of life. Some 200,000 die of heart disease and stroke between the ages of 35 and 64; and another 230,000 die within the first 10 years after retirement.

It is my opinion that this very aggressive killer of mankind can be harnessed and tamed. You don't have to become a statistic! You don't have to suffer from heart disease!

Quotation From Dr. Passwater

I feel that in order to set the tone of this booklet properly, a very good friend Richard Passwater, Ph.D., should be quoted:

Only in 1974 was the actual cause of heart disease, America's leading cause of premature death, determined. A little more than a year later, the studies pinpointing the cause were confirmed.

Many will be surprised to hear that dietary cholesterol was not found to be the culprit. *It is now believed, as a result of studies by Dr. Earl P. Benditt (of the University of Washington School of Medicine, Seattle), that the cholesterol found in the arteries at the site of the plaques (deposits) that cause heart disease is an end product of the cellular deterioration that produced the narrowed arteries (called atherosclerosis), not the cause.*

The majority of recent books on the prevention of heart disease promote the avoidance of cholesterol. Yet, no matter how carefully you follow the low-cholesterol diets, no matter how many eggs or pats of butter or glasses of milk you have dropped from your diet, you still have a 50 percent chance of dying prematurely from a heart attack. The reason for this bad news is simply that cholesterol is not the cause of heart disease.

To get heart disease, one does not have to seriously overdo one of the real risk factors; that is, sedentary lifestyle, unbalanced nutrition, high blood pressure, smoking, immoderate stress or calorie imbalance. In fact, many who do seriously overdo on one factor (and only one factor) don't get heart disease at all. Overdoing alone can be compensated for by a healthy body, or can lead to a mild form of heart disease free of clinical symptoms or problems.

But invariably when two or more real risk factors are slightly abused, heart disease will occur. And the abuses may be so slight as to be considered normal living. For example, you can avoid exercise completely, yet follow all other heart-health guidelines to the hilt and not develop premature heart disease. But if your diet is less than perfect and you don't exercise quite enough, then it's no longer a question of whether you will get heart disease, but how seriously and when. And this is the case for most Americans.

STICKY BLOOD

We can survive atherosclerosis (the deposits in the arteries that lead to narrowed arteries and increased risk of clot formation) if our blood remains slippery (as a result of sound nutrition) or if we increase the artery diameter (as a result of exercise). But if we have arteries narrowed by deposits and sticky blood, then heart disease becomes fatal. The good news is that we need only slight changes to achieve total protection against heart disease.

Most Americans have been just a little too casual in too many areas of heart-disease risk. We haven't been seriously overdoing any one risk factor and we feel that being a little lax here and there won't hurt. After all, we have cut back on eggs and butter, added a pat of margarine, and usually exercise a little every day and more on weekends.

The bad news is that too many people have cholesterol-phobia, (the needless and unfounded fear of dietary cholesterol) and their nutrition has suffered because of it. They believe that a pat of margarine and an egg substitute will protect them from heart disease. This belief detracts from a realistic approach to the prevention of heart disease. It is not the public's fault. Many are doing their best. ***But they have been misled.***

Originally physicians and scientists viewed the cholesterol deposits that accumulate in arteries as being caused by too much cholesterol in the blood. And many went even further to reason that the excess blood cholesterol came from eating too much cholesterol in our food. Even though the famous Framingham study proved this notion wrong in 1970, the myth has continued to have popular support. A few tests in the late 1950's and early 1960's at first appeared to confirm the apparent obviousness of the cholesterol-cause theory. Then better controlled and properly conducted experiments in the late 1960's and early 1970's disproved both links to heart disease.

Each of the following studies has shown that low-cholesterol diets don't reduce heart disease:

- *The St. Mary's Hospital Trial (1965)*
- *The London Research Committee Trial (1965)*
- *The Norwegian Trial (1966)*
- *The Anti-Coronary Club Trial (1965)*
- *The London Medical Research Council Trial (1968)*
- *The National Diet Heart Study (1968)*
- *The Finnish Mental Hospital Trial (1968)*
- *The Los Angeles Veteran's Trial (1968)*

- *The Framingham Study (1970)*
- *The Ireland-Boston Heart Study (1970)*
- *The St. Vincent's Hospital Trial (1973)*
- *The Diet and Coronary Heart Disease Study in England (1974)*
- *The Edinburgh-Stockholm Study (1975)*
- *The Minnesota Study (1975)*
- *The UCLA Study (1975)*
- *The Honolulu-Japanese Study (1975)*
- *Additionally, the Coronary Drug Project in 1974 showed that drugs that reduced blood cholesterol were of no value in preventing heart disease.*

Yet we hear little of these studies. (Ed. Note: If the truth in these studies were published and widely read and understood, the sale of polyunsaturated oils and margarines would be practically non-existent. How many times a day are you brain washed by an advertisement touting the low or non-cholesterol content of a food? The correction of the cholesterol-phobia would create great problems for the sale of many popular foods.)

It is now known that the arterial deposits that cause heart disease don't form as a result of high blood cholesterol levels and that eating more cholesterol doesn't raise the amount of cholesterol in your blood. (end of quote)

If Not Cholesterol, Then What Does...?

If cholesterol is really not the cause of our most deadly killer, then what is? Research which explains and documents what really happens was completed by the University of Washington and John Hopkins School of Medicine. But before we get into that research let's take a look at some of the simple facts that give foundation to that research.

a. The concept that cholesterol is not the cause of atherosclerosis is further strengthened by a simple observation: "Atherosclerosis never occurs in veins but only in the arteries." Since a laboratory technician draws blood from a vein when he checks your cholesterol, it would be quite obvious that the amount of cholesterol in the veins is similar to that in the arteries (which is born out by what we know about the circulation of blood and its contents). If this is accepted, then why do we have atherosclerosis only in the arteries?

b. A little simple anatomy course will give us a clue. It is an essential fact that the walls of veins are made up of two major layers and the walls of arteries are made up of three layers. Both arteries and veins have a similar outer and inner layer - the outer layer being more protective and the inner layer being very slippery so that the blood can flow smoothly. The muscular layer found sandwiched between the outer and inner layers in the artery allows for expansion and contraction as the heart beats, expelling blood in waves. This muscular layer also allows the constriction of the blood vessels when the "fight or flight" mechanism is activated by some kind of stress. Such constriction increases blood pressure and forces more nutrients and oxygen into the outermost parts of the body so energy levels become very high.

FACTS

1. Plaque forms only in arteries, never in veins.

2. The same amount of cholesterol flows through the veins as it does the arteries.

3. Cholesterol is the last ingredient making up plaque.

ANATOMY OF A VEIN

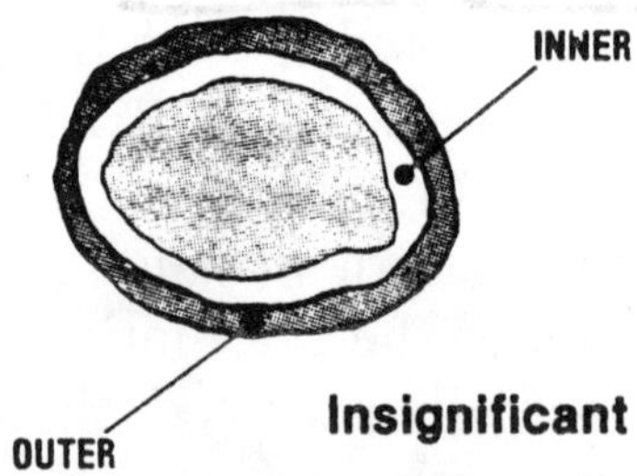

Insignificant Muscular Layer

Figure 2.

ANATOMY OF AN ARTERY

An ARTERY has 3 layers. . .

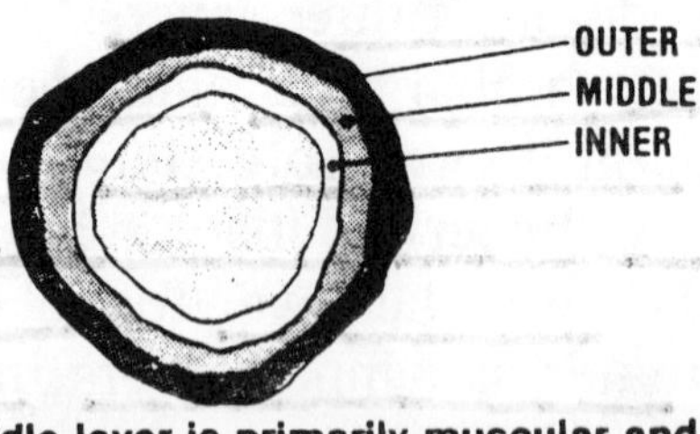

The middle layer is primarily muscular and is used by the body under stress to tighten the blood vessel thus increasing blood pressure which increases the nutrient availability, flow of oxygen, etc.

Figure 3.

THE BEGINNING

The muscular layer found in the artery may be (is) the place where cardiovascular disease begins, particularly atherosclerosis which is the lumping and plaque formation in the blood vessel. It is possible to cause changes in the cells making up this muscular layer which will result in cell division that is similar to that found in tumor formation. What is the stimulating or aggravating factor that causes normal cells to change their life style and begin to abnormally duplicate? I sincerely believe it is the **free radical**, which is an unbalanced electron acting like a chemical buzz bomb. It will penetrate a cell, alter its DNA pattern in the nucleus and open the pathway for mutation and duplication to occur.

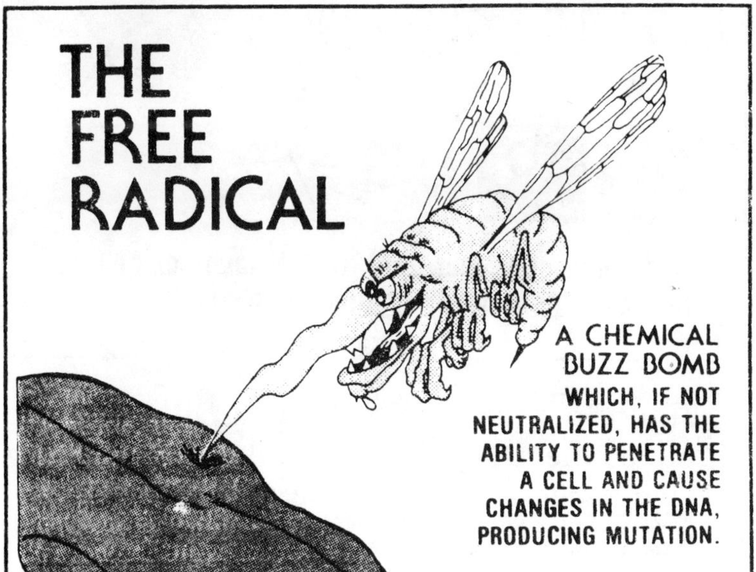

Figure 4.

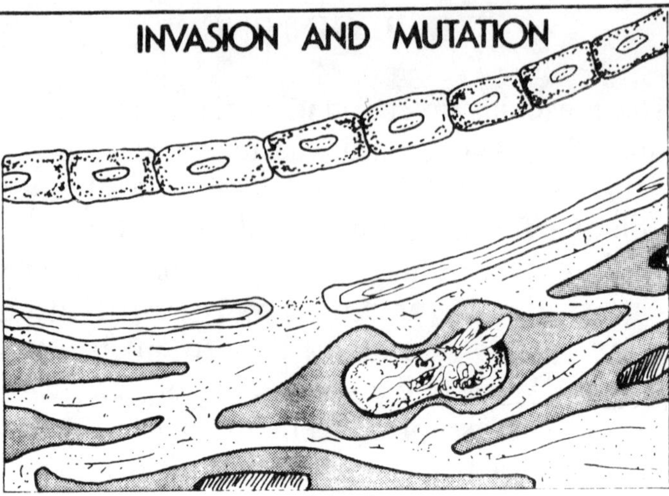

Figure 5

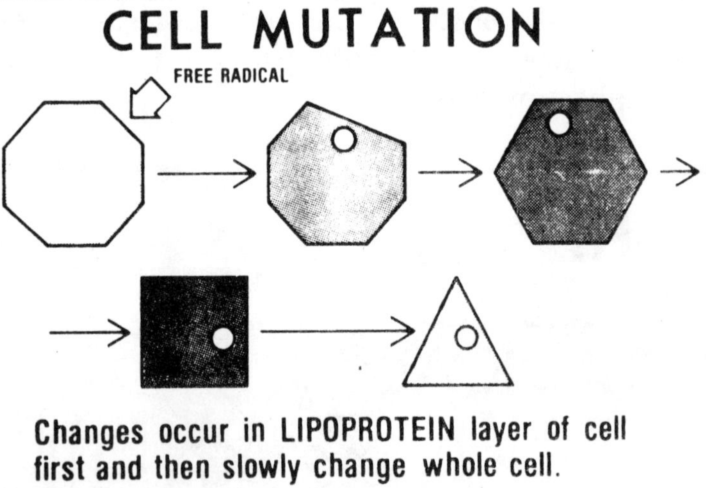

Figure 6.

Figure 6 demonstrates how a cell might be invaded, the DNA altered and the cell going through changes which still leave it alive, but no longer under the control of the signals which prevent uncontrolled duplication. Figures 7, 8 and 9 demonstrate what happens when cells begin to multiply without control.

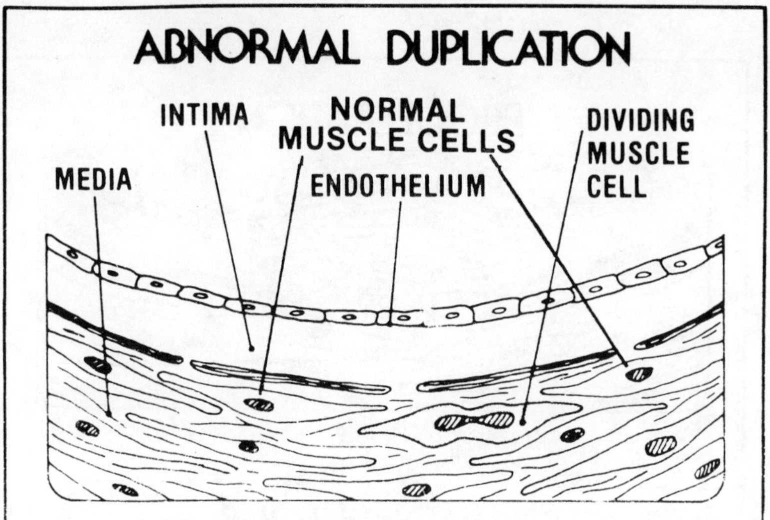

Figure 7.

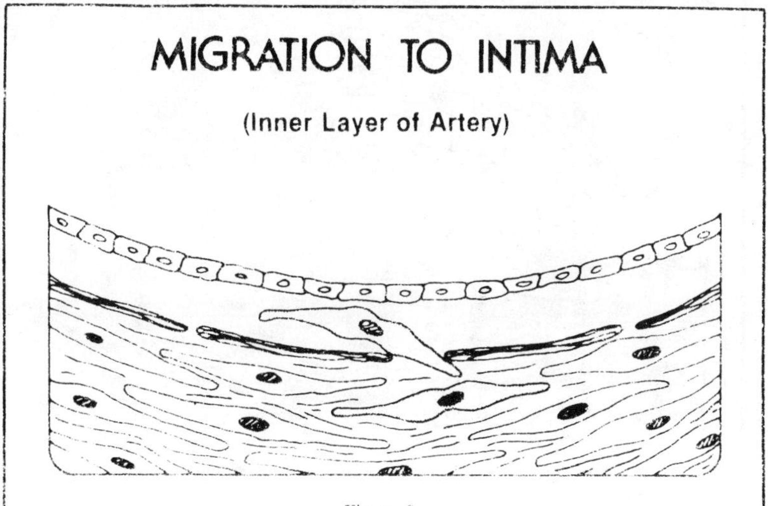

Figure 8.

As the first mutated muscle cell begins its duplication, the duplicate cell will move toward the inner lining of the artery. As these accumulate, a lump or bump will form under the single cell thick, inner layer of the artery.

PROLIFERATION

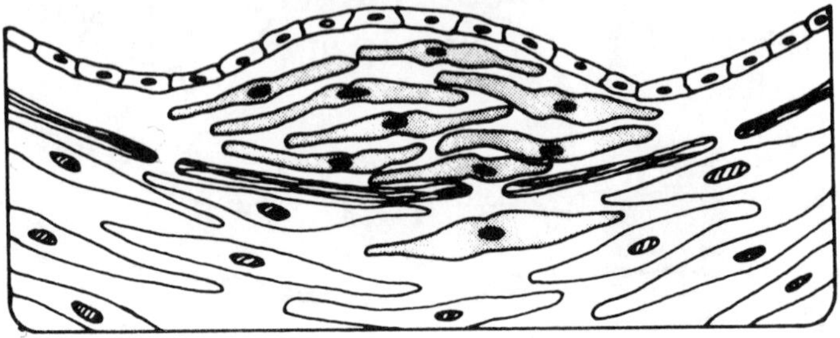

Figure 9.

LUMPY PLAQUE

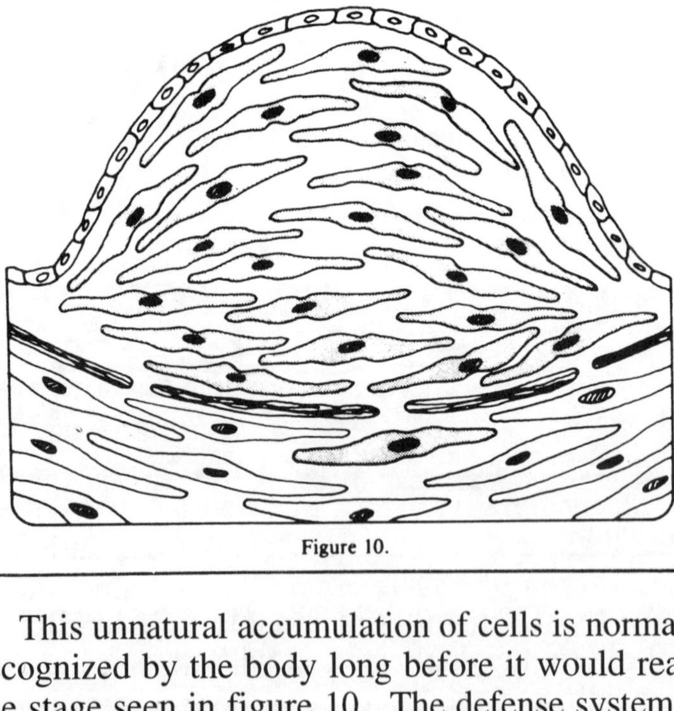

Figure 10.

This unnatural accumulation of cells is normally recognized by the body long before it would reach the stage seen in figure 10. The defense system of the body (the immune system) will create antibodies to literally destroy these abnormal cells.

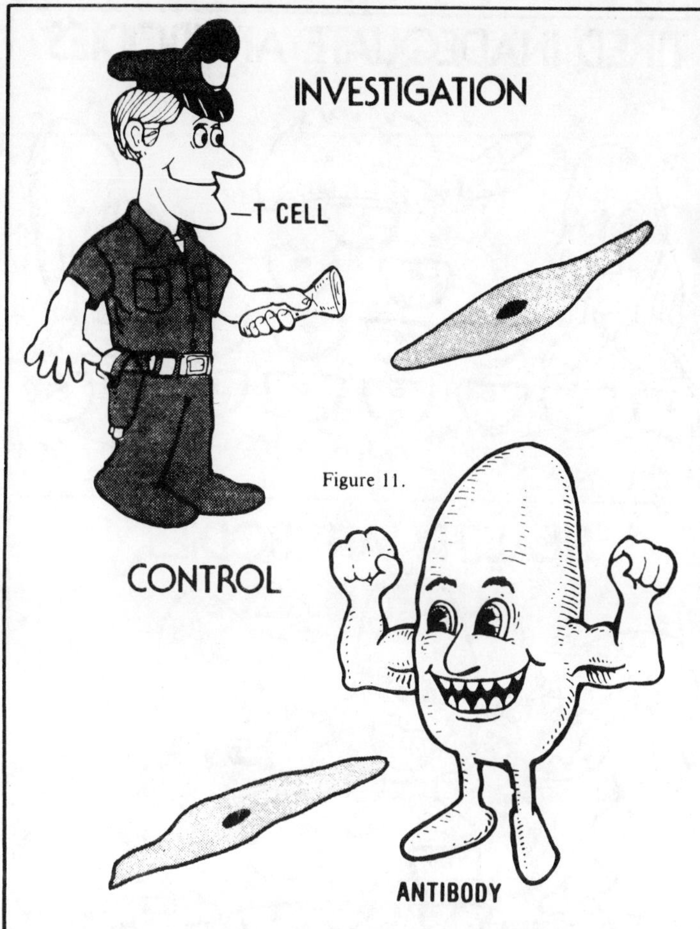

Figure 11.

Figure 12.

T Cells These thymus originated cells act as if they were a surveillance crew, constantly looking for abnormal intruders. Once an intruder is found, the T cell literally takes a picture of it and returns to the thymus with an order for a specific antibody. Once that antibody is created it is immediately instructed to go to the site where the intruder is and destroy him. If enough strong antibodies are produced the intruder is soon obliterated and no harm is done. But if our immune system is deficient, the intruder may be able to survive as we

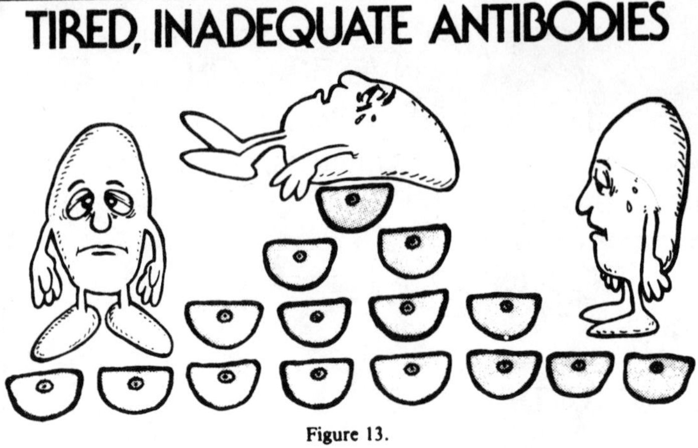

Figure 13.

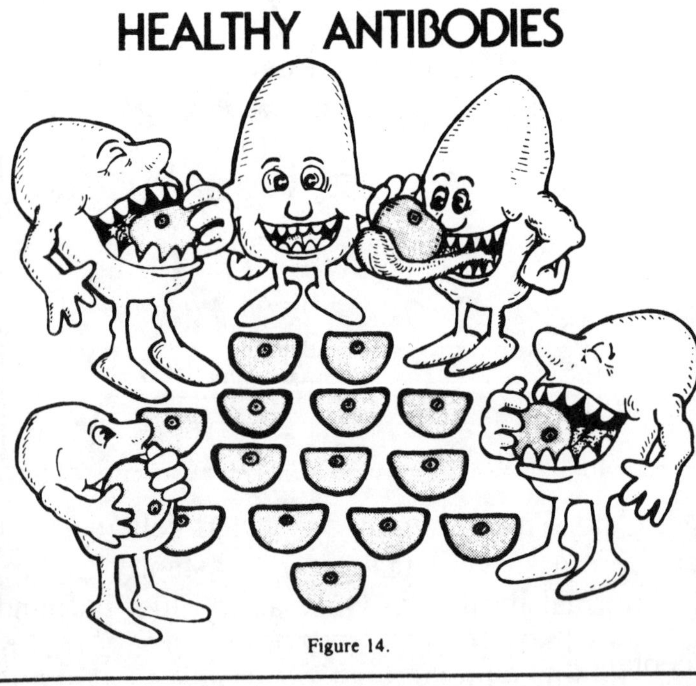

Figure 14.

see in figure 13 and multiply in mathematical progression. Most scientists are of the opinion that the foregoing process goes on constantly and the ability of the body to produce antibodies determines our susceptibility to diseases such as atherosclerosis and cancer.

HOW ABOUT PREVENTION?

In order to understand proper prevention we should investigate the chemical invader that started all this problem - the free radical. This chemical "buzz bomb" is formed by a variety of circumstances - most of which can be easily avoided.

WHERE DO WE GET FREE RADICALS?

1. Smoking - from the tars in the tobacco, not from the nicotine.
2. Consumption of unsaturated oils, particularly rancid ones.
3. Inhalation of toxic chemicals such as carbon tetrachloride, carbon monoxide, etc.
4. Constipation which releases methyl cholanthrene into the blood stream.
5. Use of chemical additives. (Nitrite + Amine = Nitrosamines,
6. Exposure to radiation. (X-rays, etc.)
7. Chlorinated water produces chloroform.

Smoking may have been demonstrated to be one of the greatest causes of heart disease and cancer known. The sad news about that is the social acceptance of this addiction which can be harder to break than that of alcohol or other addictive drugs. A real mental incentive (such as: you will die if you don't quit) or hypnotherapy or a temporary switch of dependence to another non-addicting drug, phenydantoin, may all be necessary to get this out of your life.

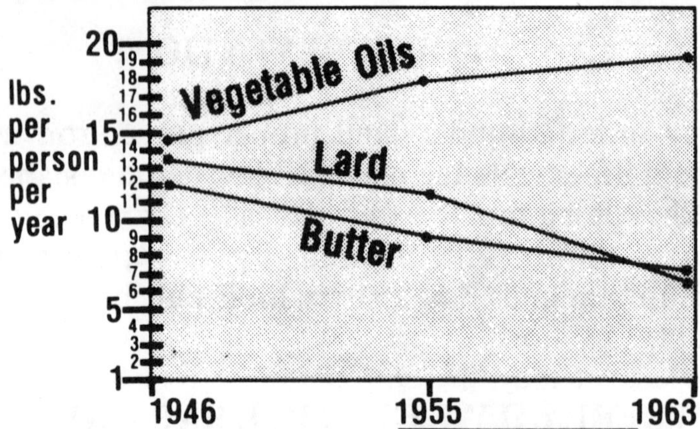

	1946	1955	1963
TOTAL ANIMAL FAT	22.3	19.1	13.3
TOTAL VEGETABLE OIL	14.4	17.7	19.0

Figure 16.

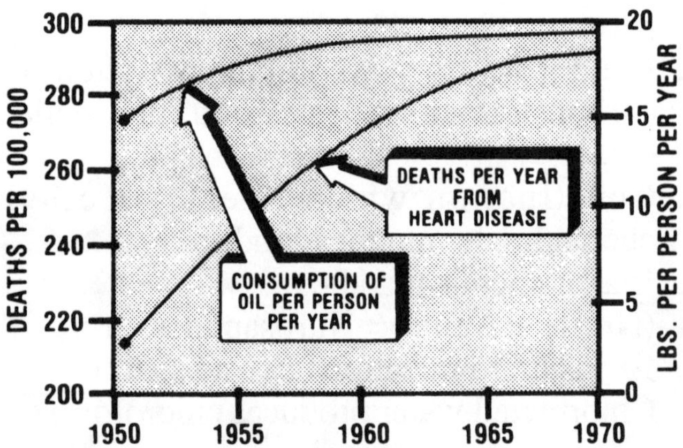

Figure 17.

Polyunsaturated oils have so long been touted as a "health food" that it is difficult to realize how dangerous a rancid oil really is. Figures 16 and 17 may help you to get a visual impression as to the correlation between heart disease and the consumption of oils. Information has been presented previously regarding the extreme importance of recognizing that these highly touted oils are dangerous!

CONSTIPATION

Constipation can become a definite factor since the putrefactive bacteria which are abundant if the feces can combine with bile acids and form a powerful free radical called 3-methylcholanthrene. The longer the time before expulsion from the colon, the more of this free radical chemical is formed. It may then be absorbed into the blood stream and in the absence of adequate vitamin E, will penetrate cell walls and cause DNA mutation. The obvious corrective actions are to increase the amount of fiber and water in the diet and be sure to consume an adequate amount of vitamin E - at least 600 units daily.

CHEMICAL ADDITIVES

We are constantly bombarded with information about the dramatic increase in chemicals in our foods, water supply and the air we breathe. To a certain extent, a properly formulated food supplement can counterbalance much of the contamination and we will discuss that in detail later. Our water supply is of major concern because it is a universal part of our daily life. Very few waters anywhere in the U. S. have water which would pass EPA standards for drinkable water. This whole problem is rather thoroughly discussed in my booklet on "Water" and you may wish to inform yourself of the problem and its solution. We shall only give a recommendation that you install a very good bone charcoal filtration unit for drinking and cooking water as well as for shower and bath water.

EGGS

The popular press and almost everyone condemns eggs when they think of cholesterol. The following chart would give one great concern about the veracity of such a theory. Looking at the governmental statistics, it becomes quite obvious that as the consumption of eggs decreased, the rate of heart disease went up almost in the same inverse proportion!

	1950	1960	1970	1980
Deaths per 100,000 Coronary Heart Disease	218	278	310	380
Eggs consumed per year per person	290	230	217	210

Taking no other statistics into consideration, we could propose a theory that the more eggs you eat the less deaths there will be from coronary heart disease.

SUGAR

Sugar consumption should also come into this equation. The more sugar we ate, the more coronary heart disease we had. Since table sugar is really a very refined product that yields two simple sugars, glucose and fructose, we might consider that if an excess of sugar is consumed, considerably less of the foods which are rich in other nutrients such as vitamins, minerals, proteins, etc., will be in the diet.

	1900	1950	1970	1980
Deaths per 100,000 Coronary Heart Disease	78	218	310	380
Lbs. of sugar consumed per person per year	40	75	120	128

This parallel should not be ignored. There are several similar parallels, the drastic decline in tooth decay during war years when sugar was rationed, the rise in the incidence of "white man's" degenerative diseases in uncivilized areas when refined sugar was introduced, etc. When the ingestion of fuel (sugar) becomes the major factor in one's diet and the maintenance nutrients become the least important, then deterioration and degenerative disease are the inevitable result! It is my opinion that the more this factor is kept out of your life, the more resistance you will have to heart disease.

OTHER THEORIES

Because of the seriousness of the cardiovascular death problem, many theories have been advanced to explain this disease. Let's take a look at some of these and see how they fit into the overall picture.

Xanthine Oxidase Theory

Kurt Oster, M.D. believes that one of the major contributing factors in artery disease involves the homogenization of milk which releases the enzyme xanthine oxidase. This is a harmful enzyme to the body and can produce a lesion in the wall of the blood vessel which then starts the fibrin-protein-mineral-cholesterol accumulation which characterizes the disease.

My problem with this theory is it is proposed that the xanthine oxidase damages the inner lining of the artery. Since the inner lining of the vein is the same, why doesn't it also damage it and produce atherosclerosis in the vein? I will accept that it injures the walls of both the artery and the vein, but plaque doesn't start just because there is an injury or we would have plaque in veins!

Homocysteine Theory

This theory of the evolution of cardiovascular disease holds that homocysteine, a normal but very toxic breakdown product of methionine metabolism, is not further broken down to a useful product called cystathionine because of a lack of vitamin B-6 (pyridoxine). Homocysteine accumulation creates atherosclerosis in experimental animals but the exact steps have not been determined. It is my opinion that homocysteine acts just like a free radical in mutating a normal cell in the middle muscle layer of the artery and creates the beginning of atherosclerotic plaque.

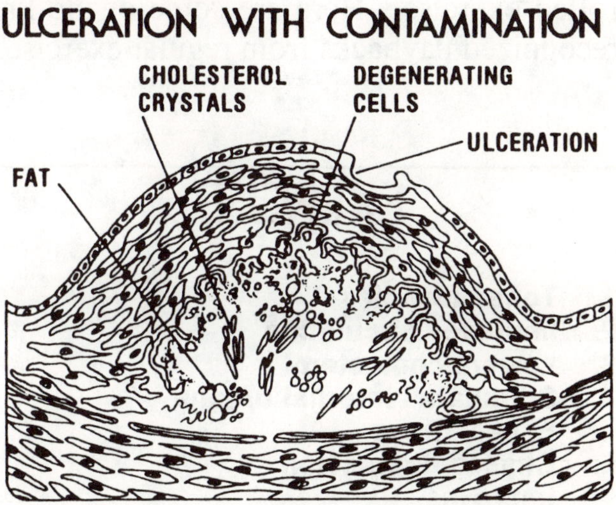

Figure 20.

In figure 20 you will see the bulge in the artery rupturing and material from the blood stream actually invading the plaque. This rupture is soon repaired by a protein constituent of the blood stream called fibrin which acts to seal off the area. Since fibrin has a fish-net like texture, it tends to trap other substances that flow by in the blood stream. This will include such materials as phospholipids, calcium, proteins, triglycerides and cholesterol. Now the formation of the inner plaque begins with evermore accumulation of materials which are bound in a cementing action by calcium. Thus, the plaque has firm consistency and is not easily dislodged.

THE EXERCISE FACTOR

More than ever we see joggers on the side of the road, stores report higher sales of exercise devices and health club memberships taking an upturn. The exercise factor in any disease process is a valid one. There are so many benefits from regular and controlled exercise. Here are some of the known and recognized paybacks from regular exercise.

EXERCISE

1. Tones muscles
2. Improves circulation
3. Lowers cholesterol
4. Stimulates internal organs
5. Eases stress
6. Chases depression
7. Improves sex
8. Promotes sleep
9. Helps you think better

---

1. Do exercise at least three times weekly.
2. Exercise should raise your pulse rate no more than 220 minus your age. Example:

   220
   – 44 yrs old
   176/minute

3. Adequate range is 120-140 beats per minute.
4. Wog (Fast walking) - Not jog
5. Do deep breathing exercises.

Figure 23.

The one fact which should be considered but is often overlooked is that exercise does not prevent nor does it remove plaque. Exercise very effectively enlarges the arteries so that it takes much more plaque to plug them up. Exercise tones muscles so that you are less likely to have a spasm of the muscular layer of the artery which is often the final cause of a coronary heart attack or stroke.

ORAL CHELATION

When I embarked on the project of determining a way to dissolve and prevent the plaquing of arteries, I was not sure of where I was going. I had a firm conviction that anything the body could do in a negative fashion, it could also reverse and create an opposite positive action.

Based upon my belief that alteration in nutrient intake produces serious changes in the body, we slowly developed a group of nutrients that were involved in helping to reduce the number of free radicals and which slowly began the dissolution of the actual plaque and prevented new plaque formation from taking place.

This formula was clinically tested on several hundred individuals, and with minor adjustments became one of the most result-producing food supplements ever produced. Establishment medicine is always criticizing nutritional approaches because of lack of "scientific protocol" which means double blind studies, etc. Our initial studies used patients with known cardiovascular problems such as reduced circulation in hands and feet, intermittent claudication (a condition in which there is severe pain in the calf of the leg upon walking), angina pectoris, history of stroke or previous heart attack. The results in a six week trial were nothing short of miraculous!

I know this sounds a bit enthusiastic, but to appreciate what I'm saying, you would have to have seen the patients who were functional cripples because of reduced circulation who became eager participants in life again. One who has such conditions should try to prove me wrong by trying the program for six weeks. If there is no improvement, then obviously I'm a charlatan and should never be listened to again. Personal testimonies from around the world are on my desk. A priest who was to have his leg amputated and could not participate in the mass any more saved his leg by using the product. A farmer who sold his farm because his doctor told him he was not ever going to be able to work again, bought his farm back after two months of using the product. His story became the basis for a feature article in a national magazine. I could go on and on.

These testimonies mean a lot to me, human suffering has been alleviated in a very small way. My only frustration is that more do not take advantage of this simple, inexpensive method of reversing deadly cardiovascular disease.

The formulation is a single product and can be used as a preventive or a therapeutic mode just by altering the number of tablets one should use. For base maintenance, one should use six tablets daily; for those with serious problems the intake should be from nine to twelve tablets daily until progress is clearly demonstrated. Since it is a very complete product, one does not have to be concerned about the use of other supplements while taking this.

THE ORAL CHELATE FORMULA

Vitamin A (Beta Carotene)	15,000 IU
Vitamin D (Fish Liver Oil)	240 IU
Vitamin E (d-alpha Toc.)	360 IU
Vitamin C (Ester C)	1800 mg
Vitamin B-1 (Thiamin HCL)	100 mg
Vitamin B-2 (Riboflavin)	30 mg
Vitamin B-6 (Pyridoxine)	90 mg
Niacin	60 mg
Pantothenic Acid	100 mg
Vitamin B-12	150 mcg
Folic Acid	240 mcg
Biotin	60 mg
Choline (Bitartrate)	450 mg
Inositol	60 mg
PABA	90 mg
Calcium (Citrate & Carbonate)	240 mg
Magnesium (Oxide)	300 mg
Iodine (Kelp)	135 mcg
Iron (Ferrous Fumerate)	4.5 mg
Copper (Gluconate)	150 mcg
Zinc (Gluconate)	15 mg
Potassium (Chloride)	240 mg
Manganese (Gluconate)	6 mg
Chromium	120 mcg
Thymus	50 mg
EPA	50 mg
Hawthorne Berry	15 mg
Selenium	120 mg
Cysteine HCL	450 mg
Methionine	120 mg
Ginko Biloba	30 mg
L-Carnitine	50 mg
Germanium	10 mg
Chondroitin Sulfate	50 mg
CoQ-10	10 mg

The above represents the content of six tablets daily, a normal maintenance level. Nine to twelve tablets per day may be indicated for some individuals.

WHY THIS FORMULA?

The body uses many different nutrient substances to destroy or neutralize the free radical and other substances which may cause injury to the body. The most important thing to remember is that the body does not use medicines to do this but it does use nutrients!

The term "oral chelation" is probably a misnomer since this formula does not chelate anything out of the body. We will explain true chelation in just a bit. However, the term "chelation" is widely known as an alternative approach to heart problems, so for convenience, I appropriated a term which is suggestive but not an actuality. This formula works in a totally different way than chelation does - but the end result is the same. It is also more convenient in certain respects since the user can take advantage of the treatment on a daily basis without leaving home.

The formulation of this product was one of the highlights of my career. It took over two years and when the first clinical trial proved successful, I was absolutely thrilled! Here are some of the reasons the formula is put together the way it is. You will note highlighted areas which indicate the important function I was looking for when formulating.

VITAMIN A Considered by some nutritionists to be one of the most important vitamins, vitamin A protects mucous membranes from damage, helps us to see better at night, and assists other nutrients in making strong gums and tooth enamel. It also **assists in selenium utilization. Vitamin A stimulates the thymus to increase in size allowing more antibody production.**

VITAMIN E A very potent antioxidant, vitamin E is often sadly lacking in the food which we consume. **As an antioxidant, it protects the body from free radicals such as superoxides, hydroxyl radicals, peroxides and lipid peroxides.**

VITAMIN C **An antioxidant** in its own right, vitamin C also helps to protect us from heavy metals, particularly lead and arsenic which can poison certain enzyme reactions in your body. Vitamin C provides considerable protection against these substances by helping to keep them in solution so they may be eliminated via the urine. Vitamin C **stimulates the production of the enzyme lipoprotein lipase (LPL) which acts as a detergent on the arterial wall.**

VITAMINS B-1, B-2, NIACIN, PANTOTHENIC ACID, B-6, PABA **These are all synergistic antioxidant nutrients which help the body in one way or another to inhibit the formation of the damaging free radicals.** Harvard University recently published a theory that heart disease was due to a lack of vitamin B-6 because without adequate supplies of this vitamin, methionine, an amino acid which is broken down in the body to cystathionine, could not break down properly and instead broke down to homocysteine, a very toxic substance. They theorized that the excess homocysteine became the actual cause of atherosclerosis and an adequate supply of vitamin B-6 would prevent the accumulation of this toxic metabolite.

CHOLINE and METHIONINE These two nutrients, one a vitamin and the other an amino acid are called lipotropics. Lipotropics are **fat metabolism assisting agents**. Choline is also involved in the neurotransmitter acetylcholine while methionine assists in many of the detoxification mechanisms in the body.

SELENIUM This mineral, essential to life in microgram doses, is rapidly incorporated into glutathione peroxidase, an antioxidant enzyme responsible for the detoxification of fatty acid peroxides, the result of the breakdown of polyunsaturated oils in the body. **Selenium is considered to be from 200 to 500 times more potent an antioxidant than vitamin E. Selenium and vitamin E are synergistic as antioxidants and inhibit or prevent the damage to tissues by free radicals which have been cited as causal factors in heart disease, atherosclerosis, arthritis and aging.**

ZINC An effective free radical inhibitor, zinc also acts to facilitate the proper utilization of vitamin A in the body. These two nutrients are a perfect example of how dependent nutrients really are, even though one may be a vitamin and the other a mineral.

CYSTEINE HYDROCHLORIDE An amino acid, cysteine protects against the damage of radiation by **terminating the free radicals** produced by ionizing radiation. The presence of adequate cysteine is also necessary to facilitate the excretion of lead from the tissues. Lead is a widespread toxic heavy metal that serves no known benefit and can cause irreversible brain damage when allowed to accumulate. Cysteine acts as a complexing agent by attaching itself to the lead and carrying it out of the body via the urine. I consider that cysteine is one of the most important ingredients in this formula.

SPLEEN and THYMUS EXTRACTS Since the immune system of the body is an important area in the control of abnormal cell formation, the use of these two nucleoprotein extracts is designed to support and assist the glands in their work. More and more evidence documents the use of nucleoprotein concentrates for glandular rejuvenation.

EPA The apparent success of the high fat and high protein diet of the Eskimos in preventing heart disease was a mystery to scientists until they determined that the oil of fish is high in a substance known as eicosopentanoic acid (EPA). **This fatty acid acts to prevent blood platelets from sticking together to form clots which would prematurely plug up arteries and produce heart attacks and/or strokes.**

HAWTHORNE BERRY If any herb has a folklore background for use in cardiovascular problems, it would be hawthorne. **Used as a cardiac tonic**, J. I. Rodale, himself a heart patient, became so enthralled with this herb that he wrote a full-length book on its background and successful use for many years in herbal medicine.

L-CARNITINE A great deal of interest has been centered on L-Carnitine recently **because of its specific action on the body's ability to utilize fats**. Carnitine has been intensely researched by professionals for several years and **its most established application has been in the treatment, or more specifically, the prevention of heart disease**. It has been found that taking an oral supplement containing L-Carnitine not only **lowers blood fat levels dramatically, but it also makes the heart stronger and healthier** and tends to normalize erratic electrocardiographic reading. Such benefits come specifically because carnitine acts to regulate the rate at which fats are burned in the body. This might lead one to speculate that carnitine might also assist in burning body fat. Such speculation has been researched and again documented as a fact although this should not be construed to mean that the casual use of carnitine will result in a trim and slim figure.

As with most products for sale, there is the real thing as well as certain imitators. Carnitine can be purchased as L-Carnitine or as dl-carnitine. Because dl-carnitine is less than one-tenth the cost of L-Carnitine, many supplement manufacturers have used the less expensive product. This is not good sense since it is quite well established that the body cannot use the d form of carnitine and, in fact, will turn away the l form as the d form begins to accumulate. Thus, you could literally be starving in a land of plenty if you had lots of d-carnitine floating around. The body couldn't use it, but because the d form is a mirror image of the l form, the body assumes there is lots of carnitine available. The bottom line is: use the L-Carnitine and leave the d-carnitine alone!

GINKO BILOBA An herbal extract from the oldest tree known to man, ginko biloba has been double-blind tested several times for its **ability to increase the oxygen content of tissue**. Each time it comes out a clear winner. Patients were able to walk farther without pain after just a few weeks of supplementation with ginko biloba. This was documented with plethysmographic readings and doppler testing of pulse volume and tone.

CoQ10 Testing has shown that **CoQ10 reduces angina and improves cardiac function**. In every test run, patients on CoQ10 had better exercise tolerance than those who had similar conditions but were not given the vitamin.

CHONDROITIN SULFATE This nutrient is a constituent of the arterial wall and **has anti-coagulant, anti-lipemic (anti-fat in blood stream) and anti-thrombogenic (prevents clots) properties**. In a particular study, the patients on chondroitin sulfate had a 10% incidence of abnormal cardiac events as compared to a 70% incidence in control patients without the chondroitin sulfate.

GERMANIUM Acclaimed as increasing the oxygen content of cells, germanium probably more accurately acts to facilitate the entry of oxygen into cells. **Anything that increases the oxygen in the cell will decrease oxygen deficit symptoms such as intermittent claudication and angina**.

A product usually is known by the effect it has on those who use it. The formula we have just discussed has become known worldwide for the benefits it has for those with cardiovascular disease. Because every function we have in the body depends upon our circulatory system, it is not surprising that many conditions which are not heart related also improve after use of this product.

CHELATION

Many have heard in recent years of a miraculous method of reducing atherosclerosis or hardened arteries by the infusion of a synthetic amino acid (disodium ethylene diamine tetracetic acid also called EDTA) into the blood stream.

Although this substance has no specific action on cholesterol or triglycerides in the atheromatous plaque, it disrupts the plaque by reducing the mineral content of the blood stream which in turn pulls calcium from the plaque to restore its own balance.

The minerals are bound by the EDTA in a form the body cannot use and eliminated via the kidneys. As calcium is pulled from the plaque, its "cementing" action is lost and the cholesterol and other substances are free to again join the blood stream.

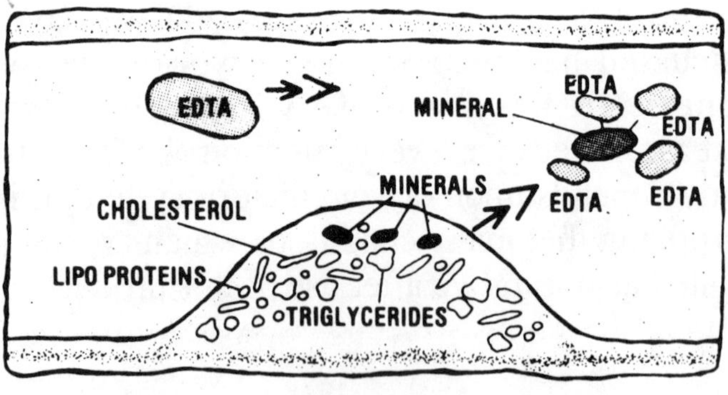

ATHEROSCLEROTIC ARTERY

Figure 22.

This cholesterol will hopefully be used by the liver to form bile and be eliminated from the body via the intestinal tract. The changes which can occur due to this plaque disruption are very dramatic in just short periods of time. Some who could not walk across the room without taking nitroglycerin for the angina pains are out playing golf within six weeks or so.

EDTA chelation technique is capable of reversing certain damage to inner walls of the artery but does not correct the basic cause. **It is not and should not be considered a preventive technique in the same sense as nutritional techniques are truly preventive, but as an emergency measure it is a life saver.**

INTRAVENOUS vs. ORAL CHELATION

Let's take a look at the mechanisms and action of the two types of chelation. It should be clearly understood that the primary purpose of both of these approaches is to assist in the elimination of our greatest killer and destroyer of normal life - namely, cardiovascular disease.

INTRAVENOUS CHELATION The intravenous infusion known as chelation therapy is definitely an effective way to reverse hardening of the arteries. Sadly, chelation therapy is not generally accepted for this purpose by the medical establishment. Most physicians who know something of the procedure erroneously believe it is too new and inadequately tested. Consequently, relatively few patients are ever made aware that a valid, specific medical treatment to unclog the arteries lies waiting to help them.

Chelation therapy is not new at all and testing has taken place by clinical and research application. It was introduced into the United States in 1948, but long before that it had been employed as a chemical medical procedure in Europe. The technique is well-recognized in all countries as effective for lead poisoning and has been used extensively in the United States for over thirty years to remove this toxic metal from the bodies of ghetto children who nibble peeling lead containing paint from apartment walls.

Chelation treatment is administered intravenously under a physician's supervision when he wishes to restore adequate blood flow through his patient's clogged arteries. The therapy is able to relieve symptoms of arterial insufficiency anywhere in the body relatively quickly.

Presently about one thousand American physicians offer chelation treatment usually to reverse or repair the effects of hardening of the arteries, including all forms of heart disease, senility, stroke and other health problems. Approximately 3.5 million intravenous infusions have been administered to over 150,000 patients. The results have been most impressive and often life saving.

How the chelation process works is no mystery. The facts are published in the medical journals, more than 1,800 articles. More than fifty physicians who administer EDTA and about 200 patients currently receiving this therapy were interviewed and a popular book describing the procedure in minute detail is available.

The chief agent used to clear the arteries is a synthetic amino acid called ethylene diamine tetra acetic acid. Since the sodium salt of EDTA is employed for unclogging the arteries, this substance is also referred to as ***disodium edetate***.

ORAL CHELATION Oral chelation is probably a misnomer since the formulation does not attach itself to or eliminate the calcium in the blood stream via the urine as does the EDTA in intravenous chelation. The term is used because the end result is the same with considerably less discomfort to the patient, not to mention considerably less cost.

In order to understand why I put the formula, which became known as the oral chelation formula, together the way it is you should know the steps that lead to the problem. With that information everything should be quite clear.

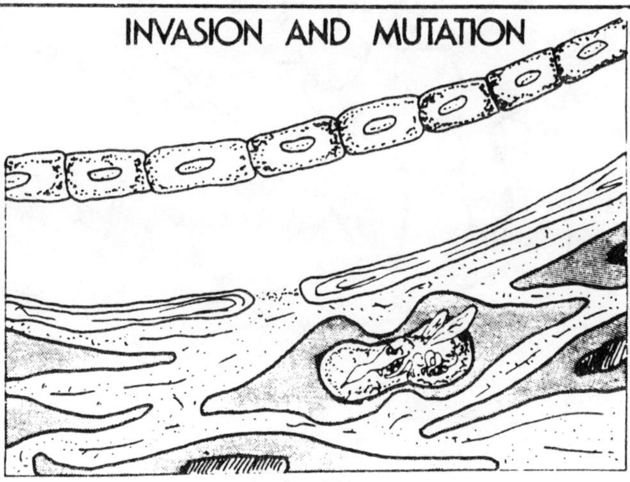

Figure 24.

In the beginning of this problem, a free radical invades a muscle cell in the middle layer of cells of the wall of an artery.

As the cell proliferation begins, T cells sound the alarm that abnormal cells are present and the thymus is called upon to produce specific antibodies to control these intruders.

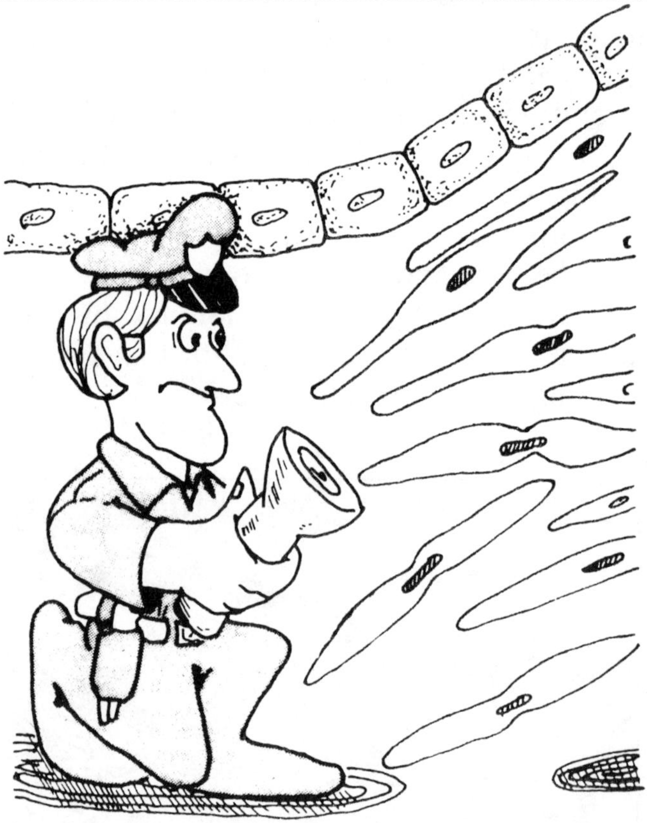

Figure 25.

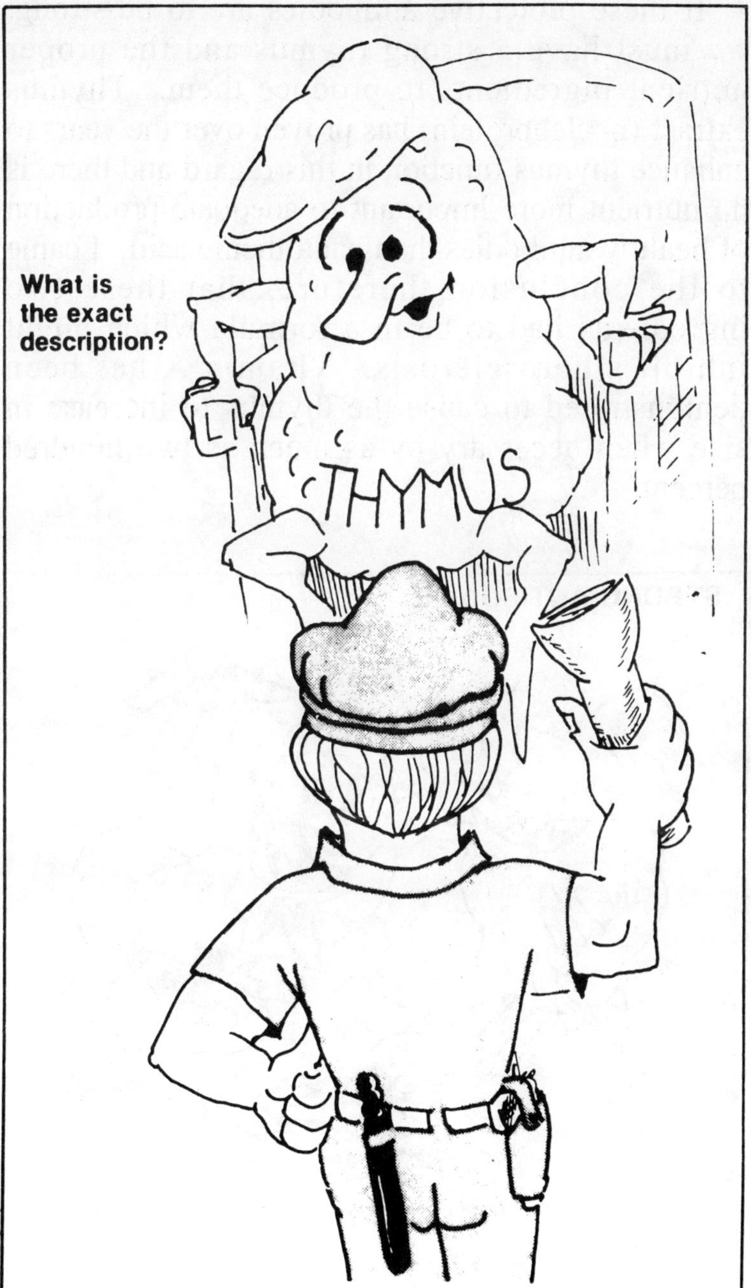

Figure 26.

If these protective antibodies are to be strong, we must have a strong thymus and the proper nutrient ingredients to produce them. Thymus extract (nucleoprotein) has proven over the years to enhance thymus function in this regard and there is no nutrient more important to adequate production of healthy antibodies than pantothenic acid. I came to the conclusion therefore, that these two ingredients had to be in a formula which might inhibit atherosclerosis. Vitamin A has been demonstrated to cause the thymus to increase in size when necessary by as much as two hundred percent.

STRONG ANTIBODIES

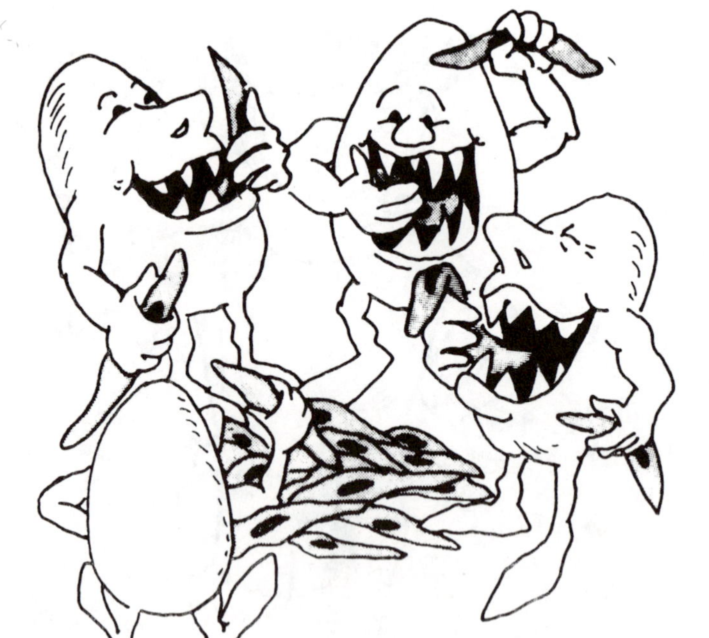

Figure 27.

But this approach only bolsters up the body's ability to resist the undesirable changes brought about by the free radical attack. Common sense will tell you that if we can prevent free radical formation, we have taken a giant step forward to eliminate atherosclerosis. The first thing to do is to avoid those things which help create the free radical:

Smoking
Consumption of unsaturated oils
Exposure to radiation
Consumption of chlorinated water
Use of chemical additives
Constipation

You must quit smoking, refuse unnecessary x-rays, eliminate unsaturated oils and margarine, filter your water to eliminate chlorine, stop using foods which contain the nitrates, nitrites and other food additives and increase the fiber in your diet to prevent constipation. It's a major change in life

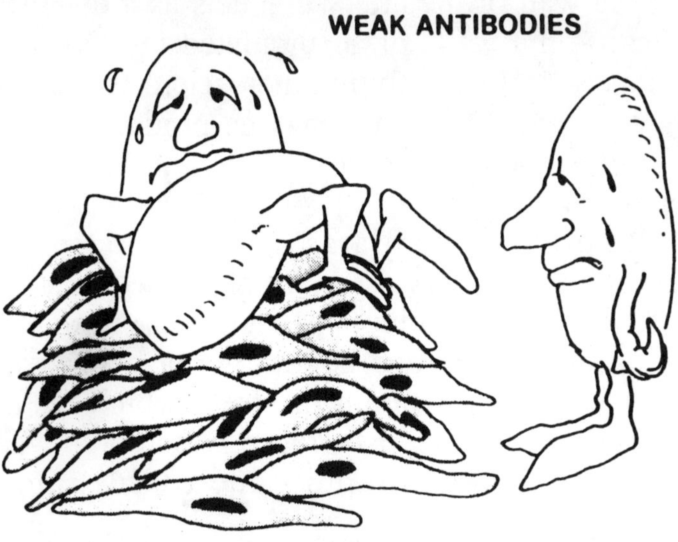

Figure 28.

style but it is also a major change in your investment plan for future health.

Another fact must be faced. If it were simply doing the few things we have enumerated here, most would quickly comply. But we must consider that the damage has already been done in most of our bodies. The records seem to indicate that atherosclerosis is epidemic in our society and the question is not who has it, but how serious is it for you. I spoke to a mortician and he indicated he had not worked on a single cadaver over the age of thirty that did not have some signs of atherosclerosis in the arterial system. Many were so far advanced that the embalming fluid did not readily flow through the plugged up arteries!

LIPOPROTEIN LIPASE

When we discuss atherosclerosis, we must discuss a little known enzyme called lipoprotein lipase or LPL for short. This enzyme is secreted from the wall of the artery and acts as a detergent to cleanse the walls of accumulated fat and other substances. Apparently in atherosclerosis, there is either not enough of this enzyme produced or the condition progresses at such a pace that it cannot keep up.

Vitamin C stimulates the production of lipoprotein lipase. Most nutritionists feel that our diets are very deficient in adequate vitamin C, particularly since our needs increase in direct proportion to the amount of stress which we are under. An interesting occurrence is displayed when vitamin C intake is rapidly increased - blood cholesterol temporarily rises because the increased LPL begins to scrub it from the walls of the artery.

And so you can see how some of the nutritional substances used in the oral chelation formula work to keep your blood vessels free of accumulating substances.

SUMMARY

The two chelation approaches, intravenous infusion of EDTA and the oral nutrient approach both are lifesavers for countless individuals. Many physicians are now opting for a combination of the two methods since they work in different fashions and by so doing find that the intravenous infusions can be cut down from a series of 30 to only 10 treatments, particularly if the intravenous formula called Ion Extractor Therapy proposed by Dr. H. Rudolph Alsleben is used.

Furthermore, by using a maintenance dose of the oral, the patient is protected for the future so he does not need to be rechelated with EDTA. Whatever form you choose, chelation therapy is a viable, positive approach to our greatest killer and deserves the consideration of both you and your doctor.

COMMON QUESTIONS

There are many questions which come up regarding the oral chelation formula. Here are some of the more frequent.

Q. How many tablets should I take?
A. The suggested dosage is six tablets daily for an interested person who wishes maintenance but for those who wish a more therapeutic effect, nine to twelve tablets daily is suggested. Please take the tablets with meals.

Q. How long should I take the product?
A. It is my opinion that you should use the product as your daily vitamin and mineral support for the rest of your life, particularly if you have any indication that your circulation may not be what you would like it to be. I like to compare it to water, if you have been deprived of it long enough for dehydration to set in and then have access to water, you will drink enthusiastically to satisfy your need. If water is accessible, you regularly drink it and do not cut back because you will once again produce the symptoms of dehydration. In the beginning you will probably use more and as you feel better it is perfectly all right to use a bit less.

Q. Why are the B complex vitamins not balanced?
A. In a product that is designed for a special purpose, it is important that certain nutrients be in higher proportion than others. There are sufficient amounts of all the B's to correct most potential deficiencies but in order to facilitate the removal of the toxic metal lead, B-1 must be

in the concentration that is listed. B-6 is commonly deficient and is very important in detoxification and free radical elimination.

Q. How about the calcium and magnesium ratio, shouldn't calcium be twice as much as magnesium instead of equal?

A. Most wholistic physicians recognize the need for more magnesium in the cardiovascular patient. It seems that a 1.5:1 ratio of calcium to magnesium is ideal but when cardiovascular conditions are present, magnesium is more important than calcium hence the 1:1 ratio in this formula.

Q. Does this product interfere with any medication I may be taking?

A. To the best of our knowledge, no. You may wish to discuss this with your physician. If you are on 1-dopa, Parkinson's disease medication, some feel that B-6 will hinder its effectiveness. Other medications, particularly the cardiac-related ones, are not interfered with by the oral chelation tablets.

Q. When is the best time to take the tablets?

A. With meals, preferably three tablets with breakfast and dinner or three tablets with each meal.

THE TIDBIT SECTION

This section is composed of tidbits of pertinent information which has been taken from journals, newspapers, magazines and other printed matter. They show the gradual outpouring of information which is totally in opposition to the "cholesterol mania" that is prevalent in our society today.

DIET AND HIGH BLOOD PRESSURE New findings indicate the usual regimen of low fat, high carbohydrate diets for hypertensive patients may be incorrect. It seems these diets cause blood insulin and sugar levels to be elevated by as much as 16%. This is a serious problem as elevated insulin and sugar are regularly associated with coronary artery disease. *(Hypertension, Vol. II, #3)*

FIBER Several new studies seem to indicate a regular high intake of soluble fiber will lower blood cholesterol as effectively as the usually recommended dosages of most drugs prescribed for this problem. Oat bran was cited as perhaps the best source of soluble fiber in relation to the amount consumed. It was noted, however, almost all fruits and vegetables provide a goodly amount of this substance. Eating oat bran decreases low-density lipoproteins (LDL's) in the blood by as much as 58%. LDL's assist in depositing cholesterol on the walls of wounded arteries, contributing to atherosclerosis, or hardening of the arteries, and subsequently heart disease. 100 grams of oat bran daily reduced overall cholesterol levels an average of 19% and since reduction of 1% in blood cholesterol is said to reduce the risk of heart attack by 2%, this results in a 38% reduction in your risk of heart attack.

BUTTER - AN ANTI-TUMOR AGENT? Because of concern about the heart disease risk posed by saturated animal fats, butter sales have been falling and margarine use increasing, notes Misuaki Sakamoto of the Nara Medical College in Japan. But butter lovers, take heart. He and his colleagues report that, at least in animals, "butter has a protecting effect" against breast tumor development. Sakamoto reported his findings at the American Oil Chemist's Society meeting.

Spontaneous lifelong breast tumor formation was compared between mice fed an ordinary diet and those fed one enriched with either 20 percent dextrin (starch gum), or 20 percent butter, or 20 percent margarine or 20 percent safflower oil. While those on the margarine and safflower oil had about the same incidence of breast tumors as mice on the ordinary diet (45%) - **only 7% on the butter diet** and 21% fed the dextrin diet developed tumors.

In rats fed the same diets as above and also exposed to a 5 mg dose of the carcinogen, DMBA, again **butter-fed animals had the lowest tumor incidence of all. Margarine-fed animals, by contrast, had the highest tumor incidence**.

ANIMAL FAT LOWERS CHOLESTEROL If the above isn't enough to make some of you animal product haters cringe, listen up - there is more that will puncture the balloon of anti-saturated fat theorists. Stearic acid, the primary saturated fat in animal fat, does not raise blood cholesterol. In fact, its cholesterol-lowering effects match or surpass that of oleic acid, the mono-unsaturated fatty acid in olive oil which is often recommended for cholesterol watchers.

In a research project, volunteers were assigned to three high-fat diets (40% of the calories were fat). One diet contained palmitic and oleic acid, a second contained stearic acid and oleic acids, and a third was primarily oleic acid.

Those on the high stearic acid diet had a 14% lower cholesterol level than those on the palmitic acid diet and a 4% lower level than those on the oleic acid diet. It was noted that foods containing reasonable portions of stearic acid do not lower the high density lipoproteins (HDL's) which are considered to be the good cholesterols while the highly unsaturated oils found in safflower for example, do lower this fraction. Many feel that although such unsaturated oils may lower cholesterol somewhat, they may be lowering the wrong factor.

All this research tends to shed some serious doubt on the heavy criticism of meat and dairy products that has been so rampant. Maybe, just like the egg, meat will regain some popularity, providing that producers leave off the hormones and medications that have a negative in the past.

BUTTER AND FATS AREN'T THE VILLAINS, SAY HEART SPECIALISTS A group of heart specialists report that low cholesterol foods do nothing to cut the risk of heart disease and in fact butter may be better than the highly advertised polyunsaturated margarines which contain unnatural fatty acids which impair the breakdown of cholesterol.

Additionally, the original molecular pattern of unsaturated vegetable oil is changed during the hydrogenation process used in making margarine and is no longer a desirable product to have floating through your blood stream.

Dr. George V. Mann of the Vanderbilt Medical School says, "No dietary therapy has been shown effective for prevention or treatment of coronary heart disease, despite a generation of propaganda. Elimination of eggs from the diet is also ineffective in cutting cholesterol levels. People would do better to go back to butter, lard and eggs."

Mann and other scientists at a symposium sponsored by the Boston University School of Medicine did not dispute the link between cholesterol in the blood and heart disease. "Lowering cholesterol in the diet doesn't mean cholesterol in the blood stream will be reduced," the specialists continued, "because it is not a problem of intake, but of the body's ability to clear cholesterol from the system."

NIACIN AND HEART DISEASE In several independent studies, niacin in the range of 2,000 mg daily was more effective in reducing cholesterol and lowering heart disease death rates than any drugs presently known. Why isn't it publicized?

CORN BETTER THAN OATS Practically everyone knows that oat fiber is very effective in reducing total cholesterol and triglycerides. Now comes corn fiber which may do the same thing, or even a little better with less caloric intake. In a study, participants were able to lower their total cholesterol levels by an average of 20% by faithfully using corn fiber daily for twelve weeks.

Triglycerides fell by 31%, an even more interesting achievement, in that none of these individuals had previously been able to lower their blood triglyceride levels with a low-fat, low-cholesterol diet. Oat bran contains 25% more calories than does corn bran, but I personally don't think that makes much difference, in that there are so few calories available in either.

EGGS, MEAT AND DAIRY LOWER CHOLESTEROL A group of men trying to reduce their moderately high blood pressure and cholesterol levels changed their diets without giving up red meat, dairy foods or eggs. The USDA's Western Human Nutrition Research Center in San Francisco said, "Go on this diet and the chances are you'll lose weight. What's more, you'll probably wind up getting more vitamins and minerals than ever before."

Average blood pressure at the beginning of the study was 135/85 and average cholesterol was 218. They did trim fats from meat, did skin chicken and in general reduced their fat intake. At the end of the study the average blood pressure was 124/79 and the average cholesterol was 185. Practically all vitamin and mineral levels in the blood stream rose, indicating that reducing the fat intake produced a more varied diet of grains, vegetables, etc.

CHOLESTEROL DOESN'T CAUSE HEART DISEASE! Scientists at the University of Southern California stated that they no longer believe that the villain in heart disease is cholesterol. Instead they are quite sure that interaction with other fats particularly the unsaturated oils and margarine creates toxic oxides which may harm the wall of the blood vessel, leading to the formation of plaque. (ed. note: The truth of this matter is that "cholesterol-mania" has resulted in one of the most lucrative markets imaginable with the endorsements of such prestigious organizations as the American Heart Association, the Heart and Lung Institute, the United States Senate Report, the American Medical Association and various other groups that were duped by some real experts. Products endorsed include the polyunsaturated oils and all the things they are used in and the margarines. One day they will be indicted as the prime cause of the epidemic of chronic degenerative disease in our society today!)

EGGS Probably no food has been more maligned during this period than that marvelous complete food, the egg. Even today, almost 90 percent of the population feel guilty every time they eat an egg. Yet an article published in Pediatrics found that animals fed "Egg Beaters" all died while those fed eggs thrived. I would hope that this makes you think before eating "unnatural" foods.

RED MEAT The eating of red meat DOES NOT increase the blood levels of cholesterol according to Dr. Bonnie Worthington-Roberts. In her study, three groups of women were put on a controlled diet plan with one group eating red meat five times a week, group 2 ate chicken and fish, and group 3 consumed only eggs and milk as a source of protein. At the end of the test, all three groups were about equal in their levels of total cholesterol and triglycerides which had not increased over the beginning levels.

BUTTER IS BETTER Butter is a close second to eggs in the maligning department. It is difficult to find butter in some supermarkets today for the stacks and stacks of margarine, a supposed healthier product. Made from unsaturated oils by a process of forcing hydrogen gas into the oil under pressure, resulting in the formation of trans-fatty acids which are very harmful to the body. When incorporated into the cell membrane phospholipid structure these acids cause the cell membrane to become excessively permeable and normal sodium-potassium and calcium-magnesium pump activity is disrupted. These trans-fatty acids also block the formation of bile salts from cholesterol in the liver thus increasing the very serum cholesterol they are supposed to lower. Polyunsaturated fat and its conversion products such as margarine were indicted as a cause of cancer in Life Sciences Journal as early as October 1976. Just remember - butter is better!

UNSATURATED OILS KILL It will come as no surprise to those of you who have read my reports or heard me lecture that the highly touted unsaturated oils have now been officially designated as "killers". The New England Journal of Medicine recently reported that if you ate butter, eggs and cheese in moderate amounts you had far less chance of a fatal heart attack than those who consumed only the vegetable oils, commonly called unsaturated oils.

IRREGULAR HEARTBEATS Magnesium can save your life if you are suffering from an irregular heartbeat. Either an injection if the condition is severe enough or oral tablets will usually help the heart restore its normal rhythm. Magnesium works in partnership with calcium and potassium to regulate the heart beat.

FISH OIL LOWERS PRESSURE - BUT FLAX OIL IS BETTER Large doses of cold water fish oil can lower mild high blood pressure as well as commonly used prescription drugs, according to an article in the New England Journal of Medicine. The participants were not too happy with the oil since it left a real fishy after taste as well as belching and slight nausea. The active ingredient in the fish oil is the omega-3 fatty acids of which the fish oils contain approximately 28 percent. Flax oil contains 54 percent omega-3s and has a bland flavor that is more acceptable to most. Dosage level is 1 ounce daily.

CHEST PAIN—HEART ATTACK??

Pain anywhere between the neck and the bottom of the ribcage, which may be dull and persistent, stabbing, burning or crushing.

START HERE

Is the pain crushing AND/OR does it radiate from the center of the chest to the jaw, neck, or arms?

YES → Is it the first time you have had such a pain?

YES → **POSSIBLE EMERGENCY Get medical help.** *This may be a HEART ATTACK*

NO → Is the pain like that of a previous heart attack?

YES → **POSSIBLE EMERGENCY Get medical help.** *This may be a HEART ATTACK*

NO → **Consult your physician. Do not delay!** *Your pain may be due to a temporary lack of oxygen in the heart. If pain persists for more than 5 minutes, get medical help at once; you may be having a mild HEART ATTACK.*

NO → Are you short of breath?

YES → Have you recently had an operation, injury, or illness that has kept you in bed?

YES → **POSSIBLE EMERGENCY Get medical help now!** *This suggests that you may have a blood clot in the lung.*

NO → Do you have a cough OR is your temperature 100°F (38°C) or above?

YES → **Call your physician now!** *These symptoms suggest the possibility of PNEUMONIA.*

NO → **Call your physician now!** *You may have a collapsed lung.*

NO → Go to next page

Continued from previous page

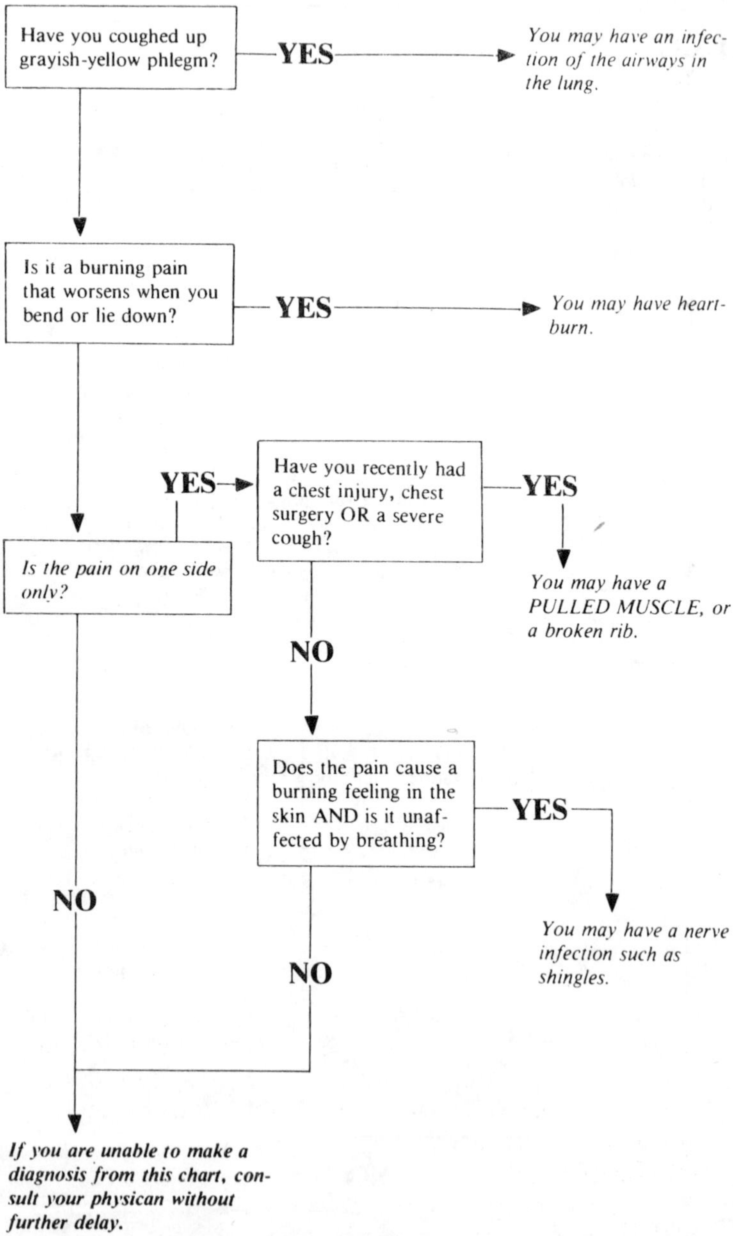

GLOSSARY

Adrenal Glands
A pair of endocrine (hormone secreting) glands that sit atop the kidneys. The inner portion of each - the adrenal medulla - secretes norepinephrine and epinephrine. Epinephrine is a heart stimulant and norepinephrine is a powerful blood vessel constrictor. The outer shell - the adrenal cortex - secretes aldosterone, cortisone, and other steroid hormones that influence the body's handling of salt, water, carbohydrates and other aspects of metabolism.

Aneurysm
A ballooning-out of the wall of a vein, an artery or the heart due to weakening of the wall by disease, traumatic injury or an abnormality present at birth.

Angina Pectoris
An episode of chest pain due to a temporary discrepancy between the supply and demand of oxygen to the heart. This may be due to low oxygen levels in the blood (from smoking or respiratory disease) to a restricted blood flow to the heart (coronary insufficiency) or to an increase in heart work beyond normal levels. Most often, angina pectoris is a chronic condition caused by a blood supply restricted by hardening and narrowing of the coronary arteries supplying the heart muscle (coronary arteriosclerosis).

An angina attack is not to be confused with a heart attack (myocardial infarction) which results from a severe and prolonged lack of oxygenated blood to a part of the heart.

Anoxia
Literally, no oxygen. This condition most frequently occurs when the blood supply (and hence the oxygen supply) to a part of the body is completely cut off. This results in the death of the affected tissue. For example, a specific area of the heart muscle may die when the blood supply has been blocked, as by a clot in the artery supplying that area.

Anticoagulant
A drug which delays clotting of the blood (coagulation). When given in cases of a blood vessel plugged up by a clot, it tends to prevent new clots from forming, or the existing clots from enlarging, but does not dissolve an existing clot. Examples are heparin and coumarin derivatives.

Aortic Insufficiency
An improper closing the valve between the aorta and the left ventricle of the heart permitting a back flow of blood.

Aortic Stenosis
A narrowing of the valve opening between the left ventricle of the heart and the large artery called the aorta. The narrowing may occur at the valve itself or slightly above or below the valve. Aortic stenosis may be the result of scar tissue forming after a rheumatic fever infection, or may have other causes.
Aortic Valve
Valve at the junction of the aorta, or large artery, and the left ventricle of the heart. Formed by three opposing cup-shaped membranes, it allows the blood to flow from the heart into the aorta and prevents a backflow.
Arrhythmia
Any variation from the normal rhythm of the heartbeat.
Arterial Blood
Oxygenated blood. The blood is oxygenated in the lungs and passes from the lungs to the left side of the heart via the pulmonary veins. It is then pumped by the left side of the heart into the arteries which carry it to all parts of the body.
Arteriosclerosis
A group of diseases characterized by thickening and loss of elasticity of artery walls. This may be due to an accumulation of fibrous tissue, fatty substances (lipids) and/or minerals.
Artery
Blood vessels which carry blood away from the heart to the various parts of the body. They usually carry oxygenated blood except for the pulmonary artery which carries unoxygenated blood from the heart to the lungs for oxygenation.
Atheroma
Also called plaque. A deposit of fatty (and other) substances in the inner lining of the artery wall, characteristic of atherosclerosis. Plural is ATHEROMATA.
Atherosclerosis
A kind of arteriosclerosis in which the inner layer of the artery wall is made thick and irregular by deposits of fatty substance. These deposits (called atheromata or plaques) project above the surface of the inner layer of the artery, and thus decrease the diameter of the internal channel of the vessel.
Atrium
Formerly "auricle". One of the two upper chambers of the heart. The right atrium receives unoxygenated blood from the body. The left atrium receives oxygenated blood from the lungs.
Blood Pressure
The force the following blood exerts against the artery walls.

Two pressures are usually measured:

1. The upper or *systolic*, pressure occurs each time the heart contracts (systole) and pumps blood into the aorta.
2. The lower, or *diastolic*, pressure occurs when the heart relaxes (diastole) and refills with blood flowing in from the large veins, the venae cavae.

The blood pressure is therefore by two numbers, with the upper one over the lower one; for example, 120/80, which is spoken as "120 over 80."

Bradycardia

Abnormally slow heart rate. Generally, anything below 60 beats per minute is considered bradycardia.

Calorie

Sometimes called large or kilocalorie. Unit used to express food energy. The amount of heat required to raise the temperature of 1 kilogram of water 1 degree Centigrade.

A high caloric diet has a prescribed caloric value above the total daily energy requirement. A low calorie diet has a prescribed caloric value below the total energy requirement.

Capillaries

The tiniest blood vessels. Capillary networks connect the arterioles and venules. Capillary walls are composed of a single layer of cells through which oxygen and nutritive materials pass out to the tissues, and carbon dioxide and waste products are admitted from the tissues into the bloodstream.

Carbon Dioxide

A waste product of chemical reactions in the cells. It passes from the cells to the blood which eventually releases it in the lungs to be breathed out.

Cardiac Arrest

Cessation of the heartbeat. As a result, blood pressure drops abruptly and the circulation of the blood ceases. Until recently, this was always fatal. Today, the heart can be stimulated to start beating again and death averted under certain circumstances.

Cardiologist

A specialist in the diagnosis and treatment of heart disease.

Cardiology

The study of the heart and its functions in health and disease.

Cardiovascular

Pertaining to the heart and blood vessels.

Carotid Arteries

The left and right common carotid arteries are the principal arteries supplying the head and neck. Each has two main branches, the external carotid artery and the internal carotid artery.

Catheter

A thin, flexible tube which can be guided into body organs. A cardiac catheter is made of woven plastic, or other material to which blood will not adhere, and is inserted into a vein or artery (usually of an arm or a leg) and gently threaded into the heart. Its progress can be watched on a fluoroscope.

Cardiac catheters can be used for diagnosis (to take samples of blood or pressure readings in the chambers of the heart) or for treatment (to implant the electrodes of a pacemaker or to administer a drug).

Cerebrovascular

Pertaining to the blood vessels in the brain.

Cholesterol

A fat-like substance found in animal tissue. In blood tests the normal level for Americans is assumed to be between 180 and 230 milligrams per 100 cc.

Circulatory

Pertaining to the heart, blood vessels, and the circulation of the blood.

Collateral Circulation

Circulation of the blood through nearby smaller vessels when a main vessel has been blocked up.

Congestive Heart Failure

"Heart failure" is a condition in which the heart is unable to pump its required amount of blood.

Heart failure is often congestive because loss of pumping power by the heart leads to congestion in the body tissues; fluid accumulates in the abdomen and legs and or in the lungs (pulmonary edema). Congestive heart failure often develops gradually over several years, although it can be acute (short and severe). It can be treated by drugs or in some cases by surgery.

Coronary Atherosclerosis

Commonly called coronary heart disease. An irregular thickening of the inner layer of the walls of the arteries which conduct blood to the heart muscle. The internal channel of these arteries (the coronaries) becomes narrowed and the blood supply to the heart muscle is reduced.

Coronary Bypass Surgery

Surgery to improve the blood supply to the heart muscle when narrowed coronary arteries reduce flow of the oxygen-containing blood which is vital to the pumping heart. This reduction in blood flow causes chest pain and leads to increased risk of heart attack. Thus, coronary bypass surgery involves constructing detours through which blood can bypass narrowed portions of coronary arteries to keep the heart muscle supplied. Veins or arteries taken from other parts of the body where they are not essential are grafted onto the heart to construct these detours.

Coronary Heart Disease

Also called coronary artery disease and ischemic heart disease. Heart ailments caused by narrowing of the coronary arteries and therefore a decreased blood supply to the heart (ischemia).

Coronary Insufficiency

A condition which occurs whenever the coronary arteries (which supply the heart muscle with blood) do not provide oxygen adequate to the needs of the pumping heart. This may produce chest pain (angina pectoris) or heart attack, or no pain may occur at all.

"*Acute* coronary insufficiency" is a term used to describe chest pain that is more severe than that of angina pectoris, but in which no heart muscle damage is done (as there would be in a heart attack).

Coronary Occlusion

An obstruction in a branch of one of the coronary arteries which hinders the flow of blood to some part of the heart muscle. This part of the heart then dies because of lack of oxygen supply. Sometimes called a coronary heart attack or simply a heart attack.

Coronary Thrombosis

Formation of a clot in a branch of one of the arteries which conduct blood to the heart muscle (coronary arteries). A form of coronary occlusion.

Cyanosis

Blueness of skin caused by insufficient oxygen in the blood. Oxygen is carried in the blood by hemoglobin, which is bright red when saturated with oxygen. When hemoglobin is not carrying oxygen, it is dark burgundy and is called reduced hemoglobin. The blueness of the skin occurs when the amount of reduced hemoglobin exceeds 5 grams per 100 cc of blood.

Diastole

In each heartbeat, the period of the relaxation of the heart. Atrial diastole is the period of relaxation of the atria or upper heart chambers. Ventricular diastole is the period of relaxation of the ventricles or lower heart chambers.

Edema

Swelling due to abnormally large amounts of fluid in the tissues of the body.

Electrocardiogram
Often referred to as ECG or EKG. A graphic record of the electric currents generated by the heart.
The word "electrocardiogram" most often refers to a resting electrocardiogram, that is the patient is lying at rest while the recording is being made. The recording can also be made during exercises.

Embolism
The blocking of a blood vessel by a clot or other substance carried in the bloodstream.

Embolus
A blood clot (or other substance such as an air bubble, fat or tumor) which drifts unattached in the bloodstream until it becomes lodged in a small vessel and obstructs circulation.

Enzyme
A complex organic substance which is capable of speeding up specific biochemical processes in the body. Enzymes are universally present in living organisms.

Epinephrine
One of the secretions of two small glands called adrenal glands located just above the kidneys. This secretion, also called adrenaline, and sometimes prepared synthetically, constricts the small blood vessels (arterioles), increases the heart rate, and raises blood pressure. It is a vasoconstrictor or vasopressor substance.

Fibrillation
A kind of cardiac arrhythmia. Uncoordinated contraction of the heart muscle occurring when the individual muscle fibers take up independent irregular contractions. ATRIAL FIBRILLATION involves very rapid, irregular contractions of the atria followed irregularly by contractions of the ventricles. This may occur suddenly and for a short time, or, if there is an existing heart disease, can become chronic. Treatment is usually by drugs and sometimes by cardioversion (brief electric shock). VENTRICULAR FIBRILLATION involves contractions of the ventricles which are irregular, haphazard and ineffective, resulting in a rapid decline of blood circulation and death. Emergency treatment may include external cardiac massage (cardiopulmonary resuscitation - CPR), electrical defibrillation (cardioversion) or drugs.

Heart Attack
The death of a portion of heart muscle which may result in disability or death of the individual, depending on how much of

the heart is damaged. A heart attack occurs when an obstruction in one of the coronary arteries prevents an adequate oxygen supply to the heart. Symptoms may be none, mild or severe and may include chest pain (sometimes radiating to the shoulder, arm, neck or jaw), nausea, cold sweat, and shortness of breath.

Doctors often refer to a heart attack in terms of the obstruction (i.e., coronary occlusion, coronary thrombosis, or simply "coronary") or of the heart muscle damage (myocardial infarction, "infarct", or "M.I."). In common usage, the term "heart attack" often incorrectly refers to irregular heartbeats or attacks of angina pectoris.

Heart Disease

A general term used to mean ailments of the heart or blood vessels. Some of these are present at birth (congenital) and are either inherited or are the result of environmental influences on the embryo as it develops in the womb. The majority of cases of heart disease, however, are acquired later in life, for example, through the development of atherosclerosis.

Heart Failure

A condition in which the heart is unable to pump the amount of blood required to maintain a normal circulation. It can be isolated to either the left or the right side of the heart, or can involve the whole heart. Heart failure can develop from many heart and circulatory disorders, especially high blood pressure (an increased resistance to blood flow in the arteries), heart attack, rheumatic heart disease and birth defects. Heart failure often leads to congestion in the body tissues; fluid accumulates in the abdomen and legs and/or in the lungs (pulmonary edema). Congestive heart failure often develops gradually over several years, although it can be acute (short and severe). It can be treated by drugs or in some cases by surgery.

Hemoglobin

The oxygen-carrying red pigment of the red blood cells (corpuscles). When it has absorbed oxygen in the lungs, it is bright red and is called oxyhemoglobin. After it has given up some of its oxygen load in the tissues, it is dark burgundy in color and is called reduced hemoglobin.

Hemorrhoids

Varices or excessively distended veins in the lower rectum and anus caused by a persistent increase in pressure within or against these veins. They are painful and often complicated by inflammation, bleeding, and clotting blood.

High Blood Pressure
An unstable or persistent elevation of blood pressure above the normal range. Uncontrolled, chronic high blood pressure strains the heart, damages arteries, and creates a greater risk of heart attack, stroke, and kidney problems. Also known as hypertension.

Hyperlipoproteinemia
The name for several types of blood-lipid disorders involving high blood levels of lipoproteins (complexes of lipids - either cholesterol or triglycerides - and certain kinds of proteins). Some types of hyperlipoproteinemia (Type II and Type IV) are associated with the premature development of atherosclerosis (hardening of the arteries) and therefore with increased risk of heart attack and stroke.

Hypertension
Commonly called high blood pressure.

Hypotension
Commonly called low blood pressure. Blood pressure below the normal range. Most commonly used to describe an acute fall in blood pressure as occurs in shock or syncope (fainting).

Hypothyroidism
A condition in which the thyroid gland is underactive, resulting in the slowing down of many of the body processes including the heart rate.

Iatrogenic Heart Disease
Literally means "caused by the doctor". A heart ailment inadvertently caused by the doctor or simply by the patient's belief that he has heart disease inferred from the manner and actions of his physician or other member of the medical team.

Intima
The innermost layer of a blood vessel (it includes the endothelium).

Ischemic Heart Disease
Also called coronary artery disease and coronary heart disease. Heart ailments caused by narrowing of the coronary arteries and therefore a decreased blood supply to the heart (ischemia).

Lipoprotein
A complex consisting of lipid (fat) and protein molecules bound together. Lipids do not dissolve in blood, but must circulate in the form of lipoproteins.

Metabolism
A general term designating all chemical changes which occur to substances within the body.

Mono-Unsaturated Fat

A fat so constituted chemically that it is capable of absorbing additional hydrogen but not as much hydrogen as polyunsaturated fat. These fats in the diet have little effect on the amount of cholesterol in the blood. An example is olive oil.

Murmur

An extra heart sound, sounding like fluid passing an obstruction, heard between the normal heart sounds.

Myocardial Infarction

The damaging and death of an area of heart muscle (myocardium) resulting from an interruption in the blood supply reaching that area.

Nitroglycerin

A drug (one of the nitrites) which relaxes the muscles in the blood vessels. Often used to relieve attacks of angina pectoris and spasm of coronary arteries. It is one of the vasodilators.

Norepinephrine

An organic compound which produces a rise in blood pressure by constricting the small blood vessels. Sometimes used in the treatment of shock. Also called noradrenalin.

Pacemaker

A small mass of specialized cells in the right atrium of the heart which gives rise to the electrical impulses that initiate contractions of the heart. Also called sinoatrial node or S-A node of Keith-Flack. Under abnormal circumstances, other cardiac tissues may assume the pacemaker role by initiating electrical impulses which stimulate contraction.

The term “artificial pacemaker” is applied to an electrical device which can substitute for a defective natural pacemaker and control the beating of the heart by a series of rhythmic electrical discharges. If the electrodes which deliver the discharges to the heart are placed on the outside of the chest, it is called an “external pacemaker”. If they are placed within the chest wall, it is called an “internal pacemaker”.

Paroxysmal Tachycardia

A period of rapid heartbeats which begins and ends suddenly.

Peripheral Vascular Disease

A term which, in its broadest sense, refers to diseases of any of the blood vessels outside of the heart and to diseases of the lymph vessels. FUNCTIONAL peripheral vascular diseases are not structural or organic in cause, but are transient and reversible. An example is Raynaud’s disease which can be triggered by cold temperatures, emotional stress, work with vibrating machinery or smoking. The term ORGANIC describes circulation disturbances which are caused by structural changes in the vessels (such as inflammation and tissue damage). An example is Buerger's disease (thromboangitis obliterans).

Phlebitis

Inflammation of a vein, often in the leg. Sometimes a blood clot is formed in the inflamed leg.

Phospholipids

One of the three major classes of lipids (fatty substances) in the blood. Unlike the other two classes - cholesterol and triglycerides - phospholipids are not known to be associated with atherosclerosis (hardening of the arteries).

Plaque

See Atheroma.

Plasma

The cell-free liquid portion of uncoagulated blood. It is different from serum which is the fluid portion of the blood obtained after coagulation.

Platelets

One of the three kinds of formed elements found in the blood. Literally "little plates", they are small, colorless, disk-shaped bodies which are involved in the formation of blood clots. Also called thrombocytes.

Polyunsaturated Fat

A fat so constituted chemically that it is capable of absorbing additional hydrogen. These fats are usually liquid oils of vegetable origin, such as corn oil or safflower oil. A diet with a high polyunsaturated fat content tends to lower the amount of cholesterol in the blood. These fats are sometimes substituted for saturated fat in a diet in an effort to lessen the hazard of fatty deposits in the blood vessels.

Prostaglandins

Hormone-like substances made from fatty acids which are found throughout the body tissues. They are thought to have important roles in tissue metabolism and blood flow, among other things.

Pulmonary Circulation

The circulation of the blood through the lungs, the flow being from the right lower chamber of the heart (right ventricle) through the lungs, back to the left upper chamber of the heart (left atrium).

Pulmonary Edema

A condition, usually acute (sudden and severe) but sometimes chronic, marked by an excess of fluid in the extravascular (outside the vessels) spaces in the lungs. It may be confined to the interstitial spaces or may appear in the alveoli (the millions of tiny air sacs in each lung). Pulmonary edema occurs most often as a complication of left ventricular failure due to ischemic heart disease, high blood pressure or disease of the aortic valve.

Pulmonary Embolism

A condition in which a blood clot (embolus), usually one formed in a vein of the leg or pelvis, breaks loose and becomes lodged in one of the arteries of the lungs. This may produce no symptoms at all or may create very serious impairment of pulmonary circulation.

Pulmonary Hypertension

High blood pressure (hypertension) in the blood vessels of the lungs. The two most common causes are chronic obstructive lung diseases (such as emphysema) and septal defects (holes in the wall which separates the left and right side of the heart).

Pulse

The expansion and contraction of an artery may be felt with the finger.

Pulse Pressure

The difference between the blood pressure in the arteries when the heart is in contraction (systole) and when it is in relaxation (diastole).

Renal Circulation

The circulation of the blood through the kidneys. Important in heart disease because of its function in the elimination of water, certain chemical elements, and waste products from the body.

Saturated Fat

A fat so constituted chemically that it is not capable of absorbing any more hydrogen. These are usually the solid fats of animal origin such as the fats in milk, butter, meat, etc. A diet high in saturated fat content tends to increase the amount of cholesterol in the blood. Sometimes these fats are restricted in the diet in an effort to lessen the hazard of fatty deposits in the blood vessels.

Sclerosis

Hardening, as in the term "arteriosclerosis", of the arteries.

Stroke

Also called cerebral vascular accident. An impeded blood supply to some part of the brain generally caused by:

1. A blood clot forming in the vessel (cerebral thrombosis).
2. A rupture of the blood vessel wall (cerebral hemorrhage).
3. A blood clot or other material from another part of the vascular system which flows to the brain and obstructs a cerebral vessel (cerebral embolism).
4. Pressure on a blood vessel, as by a tumor.

Systemic Circulation
The circulation of the blood through all parts of the body except the lungs, the flow being from the left lower chamber of the heart (left ventricle) through the body, back to the right upper chamber of the heart (right atrium).
Systole
In each heartbeat, the period of contraction of the heart. Atrial systole is the period of the contraction of the upper chambers of the heart called the atria.
Ventricular systole is the period of the contraction of the lower chambers of the heart called the ventricles.
Tachycardia
Abnormally fast heart rate. Generally, anything over 100 beats per minute is considered a tachycardia.
Thromboangitis Obliterans
Also called Buerger's disease. A disease of the blood vessels of the extremities, primarily the legs, which occurs most commonly in men and is associated with tobacco use. It is characterized by inflammation of the veins, arteries and nerves and by thrombosis in the vessels (blood clot formation). This leads to poor circulation and gangrene.
Thromboembolism
Obstruction (embolism) of a blood vessel by a blood clot (thrombus) formed elsewhere in the circulatory system and carried along by the bloodstream to plug a smaller vessel.
Thrombophlebitis
Inflammation and blood clotting in a vein.
Thrombosis
The formation or presence of a blood clot (thrombus) inside a blood vessel or cavity of the heart.
Varicose Veins
Also called "varicosities" and "varices," they are swollen veins found most frequently on the legs, especially the calves.
Vasoconstrictor
Vasoconstrictor nerves are a part of the involuntary nervous system. When these nerves are stimulated, they cause the muscles of the arterioles to contract, narrowing the arteriole passage, increasing the resistance to blood flow, and raising the blood pressure.
Vasoconstrictor agents (or vasopressors) are chemical substances which stimulate the muscles of the arterioles to contract. An example is norepinephrine (noradrenalin).

Vasodilator

Vasodilator nerves are certain nerve fibers of the involuntary nervous system which cause the muscle of the arterioles to relax, thus enlarging the arteriole passage, reducing resistance to the flow of blood, and lowering blood pressure.

Vasodilator agents are chemical compounds which cause a relaxation of the muscles of the arterioles. Examples are nitroglycerin and other nitrites, hydrazine, and many others.

Vein

Any one of a series of vessels of the vascular system which carries blood from various parts of the body back to the heart. All veins in the body conduct unoxygenated blood except the pulmonary veins which conduct freshly oxygenated blood from the lungs back to the heart.

Venous Blood

Unoxygenated blood. The blood, with hemoglobin in the reduced state, is carried by the veins from all parts of the body back to the heart and then pumped by the right side of the heart through the pulmonary artery to the lungs where it is oxygenated.

Ventricle

One of the two main pumping chambers of the heart. The left ventricle pumps oxygenated blood through the arteries to the body. The right ventricle pumps unoxygenated blood through the pulmonary artery to the lungs. Capacity of each ventricle in an adult averages 85 cc. or about 3 ounces.

CIRCULATORY DIAGRAMS

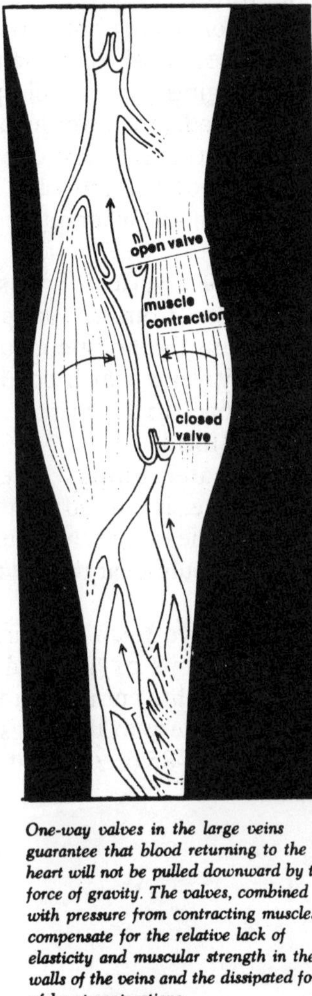

One-way valves in the large veins guarantee that blood returning to the heart will not be pulled downward by the force of gravity. The valves, combined with pressure from contracting muscles, compensate for the relative lack of elasticity and muscular strength in the walls of the veins and the dissipated force of heart contractions.

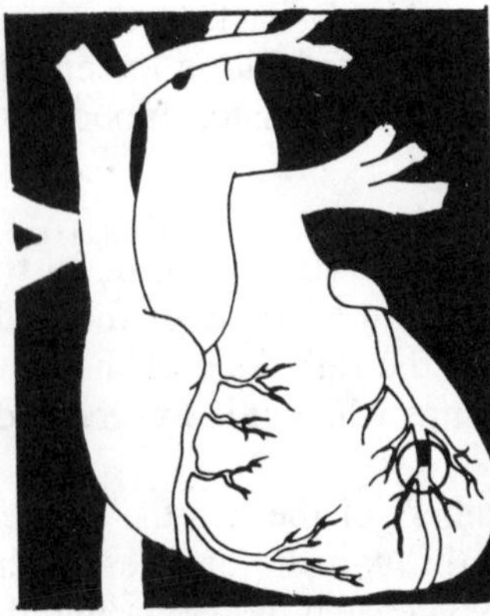

Atherosclerotic deposit in the wall of a coronary artery narrows the opening through which blood flows, reducing the supply of oxygen to the heart muscle. A blood clot trapped in the narrow opening may completely obstruct the flow and thus deprive the tissue of vital oxygen.

The right heart receives blood from the body and pumps it through the pulmonary artery to the lungs where the blood gets rid of carbon dioxide and picks up a fresh supply of oxygen. The left heart receives oxygen-rich blood from the lungs via the pulmonary veins and pumps it through the aorta to the body.

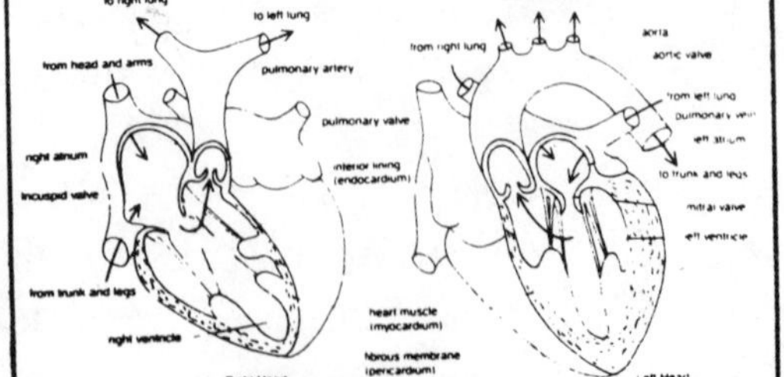

HOW THE HEART WORKS

DIET RULES FOR THE CARDIOVASCULAR PATIENT

A. REGARDING THE USE OF SALT People who use as much salt as they like may excrete nine times as much potassium, an essential mineral, as those on salt restricted diets. Actually Americans frequently consume 20 to 25 times as much salt as estimated sodium requirements recommend. If this is not counterbalanced with increased potassium intake, a borderline potassium deficiency state is easily brought about. Salt substitutes, mostly made up of potassium chloride, are often too bitter for anyone to stick with. A seasoning salt made up of 60 percent potassium and 40 percent sodium, plus some calcium and magnesium is now available and the ideal seasoning for all your foods.

B. HIGH FIBER FOODS Constipation is a natural enemy of any health recovery program. It is easy to get enough fiber if you have one bowl of whole grain cereal every breakfast and have one cupful of fruit daily. In addition, you should eat four cupfuls of vegetables per day. Since fiber requires a sufficient amount of water to do its job, we recommend that you consume at least two quarts of fluid daily.

C. REGARDING THE USE OF FATS IN THE DIET You should never use margarine, shortening or unsaturated oil. Use butter, olive oil and peanut oil in cooking.

D. REGARDING THE USE OF MEAT IN THE DIET You should consume a variety of fish, fowl, meat, dairy products, nuts and seeds. It should be understood that the requirements of B will take precedence - eat your vegetables first!

E. Processed meats such as lunch meats and hot dogs are not good food. Concentrated sugar foods should only be eaten as special treats, maybe once a week. Excessive consumption of coffee, tea or alcohol is expressly forbidden.

THE OXYGEN FACTOR

It has been my experience that everyone who has any kind of disease will have a lower total oxygen content of the blood. Another unfailing observation is that the oxygen level will come up toward normal as the patient begins to get well. From this evidence we began to use oxygen as a therapeutic modality.

Utilizing a form of liquid oxygen called magnesium peroxide can be of great benefit to anyone suffering from any disturbance in the body. This oral form of oxygen can be safely used in almost any quantity except that too much will make you a bit hyperactive.

Certainly, cardiovascular disease is the easiest disease on which to demonstrate loss of oxygen to the tissue. Lack of oxygen to the heart muscle causes angina and eventually a heart attack. Loss of oxygen supply to brain cells causes the crippling after effects of a stroke.

Oxygen also demonstrates some ability to remove plaque in the artery so you have the double benefit of greater oxygen supply as well as a therapeutic benefit.

One caution on oral liquid oxygen ingestion. For best results always use on an empty stomach. It will have little benefit if taken with food or juices.